Praise for *Wil*

T0032413

"Reading this book is like letting a trusted friend take your hand and walk with you. Alison Zak is a wise guide who shows us how to face our deepest questions about the self and others, and humans and animals. *Wild Asana* teaches us how to live and learn from and with each other in order to bring about balance both within and without. Our bodies—like the hand of a friend in our hand—will lead the way. Combining insightful stories and practical methods, this book is perfect for beginners and experienced yoginis alike. Let its seed go wild in you so you may bloom with beauty and well-being."

—CASSIE PREMO STEELE, PhD, author of *Earth Joy Writing*

"*Wild Asana* is a song for the spirit. Alison's own story—one of interconnection and reverence for nature and other beings—is told in a way that makes yoga and deep connection accessible for all of us. The world needs this book now, and I am grateful to Alison for sharing her beautiful words and opening our hearts."

—BETH ALLGOOD, president of OneNature

"One definition of yoga is 'connection.' In this unique and thoughtful book, Alison Zak muses beautifully on the connections between humans, animals, and the planet—all through the lens of yoga. Readers will finish the book feeling more connected to themselves, their practice, and the world. It's a worthy addition to any thinker's library."

—SAGE ROUNTREE, PhD, E-RYT 500, author of *Everyday Yoga*
and coauthor of *Teaching Yoga Beyond the Poses*

"Yoga is an ancient mystical practice that has become a mostly indoor pursuit in the modern world. In this delightful book, Alison reminds us of hatha yoga's wild roots, in fact she 'rewilds' the practice, bringing her love of animals and the 'living earth' so that we can reclaim the primal, untamed energy that gave rise to the practice that has swept the world and become a part of everyday life. What a beautiful invitation to seek the wisdom and the power that our 'more than human' relatives have to share and own what is truly Yoga."

—MICAH MORTALI, author of *Rewilding*

"As a naturalist and wildlife conservationist who's always been curious about yoga, Zak's book offered me the perfect entry point to delve into the practice through my love of animals and commitment to conservation."

—DAVID MIZEJEWSKI, naturalist and TV host, National Wildlife Federation

"*Wild Asana* is inviting, imaginative, and restoring, reestablishing our ancient connection with all of life in an original, welcoming, freeing way. A great way to celebrate and honor our bodies and our world!"

—SY MONTGOMERY, author of *How to Be a Good Creature*

"Mix one part lore, one part science, a draught of personal essay, and a dash of yoga, then stir in a bit of mysticism. The result is *Wild Asana*, a delightful concoction that will help you breathe into the magic and mystery of the natural world."

—MAIA TOLL, award-winning author of the *Wild Wisdom* series

"*Wild Asana* uses storytelling, personal experience, and research to uncover the tapestry of animal kinship, nature, and the roots of yoga. Equal parts scientific, scholarly, and spiritual, [the book] brings us closer to both our divine and animal natures, lovingly detailing their interdependence, and the ways in which the ancient art of yoga intertwines with our humanity. A longtime Iyengar practitioner and animal advocate myself, I applaud this book."

—SARAH C. BEASLEY, award-winning author of *Kindness for All Creatures*

"With every page, I felt *Wild Asana* attuning me to the living connection between the yoga postures I love, the animals they honor, and the heart of humanity. In her paean to the interdependence of the human spirit and the natural world, Alison Zak flows effortlessly between science, poetry, myth, and memoir—reminding us that true yogis are both naturalists and mystics."

—ANNE CUSHMAN, author of *The Mama Sutra* and *Moving into Meditation*

"*Wild Asana* is a deeply compassionate and playful exploration of how we are still animal and connected to other species in the animal kingdom through asana and nature. It is a profoundly impactful journey that supports a shift in your perspective and includes practices that reanimate the body and spirit, working toward the goal of reweaving humans back into nature. Beautifully written and thoughtfully designed, this book is a warm and bright companion on the journey back to your wild nature."

—EILA KUNDRIE CARRICO, author of *The Other Side of the River*

"Part natural history, part memoir, part spiritual reflection, *Wild Asana* is a delight for the body and mind. A central theme is the importance of humans' connection with and ethical responsibility toward the natural world. With each chapter devoted to a different animal/pose, Zak elegantly weaves together personal experience and reflection and scientific research to illustrate how yoga constitutes a pathway through which we can realize our connections with other animals, or 'beyond-human beings.' At times serious, at times humorous, Zak's poetic-like prose is welcoming and thought provoking, resulting in a read to be enjoyed by all, yogi or not."

—DR. ERIN P. RILEY, professor of anthropology at San Diego State University

WILD

ASANA

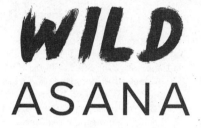

WILD
ASANA

Animals, Yoga, and Connecting Our Practice to the Natural World

ALISON ZAK

North Atlantic Books

Huichin, unceded Ohlone land
aka Berkeley, California

Published by
North Atlantic Books
Huichin, unceded Ohlone land
aka Berkeley, California

Cover art and design by Jasmine Hromjak
Illustrations by Jasmine Hromjak
Book design by Happenstance Type-O-Rama

Printed in the United States of America

Wild Asana: Animals, Yoga, and Connecting Our Practice to the Natural World is sponsored and published by North Atlantic Books, an educational nonprofit based in the unceded Ohlone land Huichin (*aka* Berkeley, CA) that collaborates with partners to develop cross-cultural perspectives; nurture holistic views of art, science, the humanities, and healing; and seed personal and global transformation by publishing work on the relationship of body, spirit, and nature.

North Atlantic Books's publications are distributed to the US trade and internationally by Penguin Random House Publisher Services. For further information, visit our website at www .northatlanticbooks.com.

MEDICAL DISCLAIMER: The following information is intended for general information purposes only. Individuals should always see their health care provider before administering any suggestions made in this book. Any application of the material set forth in the following pages is at the reader's discretion and is their sole responsibility.

Library of Congress Cataloging-in-Publication Data

Names: Zak, Alison, author.
Title: Wild Asana : animals, yoga, and connecting our practice to the
    natural world / Alison Zak.
Description: Berkeley, California : North Atlantic Books, [2023] | Includes
    bibliographical references and index. | Summary: "An embodied
    exploration of the animals that inspire familiar yoga poses, drawing on
    wildlife science, anthropology, Hindu mythology, Eastern philosophy, and
    personal stories"— Provided by publisher.
Identifiers: LCCN 2022049828 (print) | LCCN 2022049829 (ebook) | ISBN
    9781623178079 (trade paperback) | ISBN 9781623178086 (ebook)
Subjects: LCSH: Yoga. | Human-animal relationships.
Classification: LCC RA781.67 .Z35 2023 (print) | LCC RA781.67 (ebook) |
    DDC 613.7/046—dc23/eng/20230111
LC record available at https://lccn.loc.gov/2022049828
LC ebook record available at https://lccn.loc.gov/2022049829

1 2 3 4 5 6 7 8 9 KPC 27 26 25 24 23

To my nephew,
Alley Muhammad Zak

Contents

Note about language: Sanskrit terms are included without diacritical marks and transliterated to favor common English pronunciation and pluralization for readability. Due to the nature of Sanskrit and its evolving use in yoga, some of the animal names and corresponding pose names differ. I write about animals as beings instead of things (who versus that) and randomly assign gendered pronouns if their biological sex is unknown (he/she/they versus it). I look forward to the day when we embrace Robin Wall Kimmerer's suggestion to use the pronoun *ki* to revere, through language, the kinship we share with all living beings.

"GOOD MORNING SUN!"

We're pondside on a warm, July morning. Children greet the sun with enthusiastic salutations; first with their voices, then with their bodies. The kids flow through mountain, praying mantis, oak tree, and beaver lodge pose, reaching fingers to the sky then down toward the earth where pant legs are tucked into socks. They balance and sway in the breeze. They howl in downward-facing coyote, scream like bobcats, flaunt their antlers in buck pose, and writhe like hognose snakes. For a few moments each morning of summer camp, before the children spend the day hiking, playing games, and learning outside, they are joyously animal.

When you read the word *animal,* what critter arises in your mind? We are eager to conjure images of any animal but ourselves. From polar bears to water bears and fire ants to cormorants, we share this planet with some amazing creatures. We observe and interact with many of them. Whether or not we notice other animals, mimic their forms in a yoga class, or learn how to survive in this world from their behaviors as our ancestors did, they exist and they are sacred. They do not need human animals to legitimize their being here. It is comforting to me that I can write this book for one animal species to read while millions of others care nothing about it, except for the worms, many generations into the future, who might feast upon the pages in your hands. We don't all read, but we do all need each other to survive.

Let's discuss a few things, dear reader. First, I encourage you not to get hung up on the term *species.* I use it—I did in the previous paragraph.

I must. I am part scientist. But I am also part mystic who rejects the term as another obstacle impeding unity. *Species* is a concept invented and used by people to make sense of the natural world. Yet Darwin himself wrote, "I look at the term species as one arbitrarily given for the sake of convenience."[1] Living things evolve and change over time due to many factors, but there is never one moment during which a creature stops being one species and starts being another. Just as there is never one point at which a child suddenly becomes an adult; yet, numerical age and our perception of linear time are useful social constructs. It is the same with biological species. These boundaries are arbitrarily imposed by scientists who group things by similarity in order to function. This is not a problem or a criticism. It is simply a fact.

The most detailed categorization many scientists use to understand living things is *species* or *subspecies.* Mystics, yogis, buddhas, and some scientists, too, choose to focus instead on the individual as the smallest possible unit. An individual animal is physically (if not energetically) discrete, while a species is not. We are forced to shove the individual into a species category, even when it is not necessarily the reality that the individual experiences. You could say, "This invasive python should live in Southeast Asia, not Florida," but that is not the reality of the individual snake hatched and living the only life he knows in the steamy, swampy Everglades. Although *species* is the lowest level of Latin taxonomy, it is often still too broad to manage the ways in which we relate to other beings. So, don't remain too attached to King Philip's spaghetti shenanigans (or whatever mnemonic you learned in high school to remember the Linnaean taxonomic order: kingdom, phylum, class, order, family, genus, species). The way we currently classify life is like anything else in science—working for us imperfectly for now but bound to change; hallelujah!

You will also find that, because my use of the term *species* is a little fuzzy, there are doves in the pigeon chapter, alligators in the crocodile chapter, and rattlesnakes in the cobra chapter. I have not been lucky enough to encounter a cobra in the wild (yet) and neither have many of my yoga students here in the United States. I invite you to embrace this chaos and broaden the boundaries of your brain's current classification system while simultaneously reflecting on your own relationships with locally relevant animals and landscapes.

Speaking of what is working for us now, let's define another term. Assume that when I use the word *animal*, humans are included. When I distinguish human animals from all the other wonderful beings in kingdom Animalia, I may also use the term *beyond-human beings*. *Beyond* in this case does not imply superior; rather, it encourages us to open our minds and expand our understanding of shared experiences, those that challenge us as they inspire more profound connection. *Beyond-human being* is a little clunky, yes, but less human-centric than alternatives such as *other-than-human* and *nonhuman*, both of which perpetuate the boundary between human and everything-else-other-than. It still uses our species as the reference point, but in a less dichotomy-enforcing way. The use of *beyond-human being* also allows for the inclusion of non-animal but arguably living things such as trees, mountains, and rivers. And while this book is about animals and *asana* (the physical, postural practice of yoga), I intentionally leave this door wide open to suit your personal relationship with nature. In short, no existing term is perfect, so I use those that are good enough and clear enough.

Why beyond-human *being*? *Being* is both a noun and a verb: a human being versus human *being*. With audacity we lump persons, places, and things together into the same mundane package. Me, the Himalayas, a glass jar. Whether you believe other animals are people or things, we're all the same: we're nouns. That's how language always reminds me of the sacred. Silly little elementary school Alison was led to believe that nouns were the easiest parts of speech to master. But isn't that how it goes? The simplest thing is actually the most complex and the most important. Like breathing.

We cannot contemplate animals for long before we are forced to grapple with the concept of *anthropomorphism*, the attribution of human characteristics to beyond-human beings. It used to be a grave sin, especially in the sciences, to anthropomorphize. For example, I was once tasked with developing an ethogram, a catalog of behaviors, for a captive group of ring-tailed lemurs. Every inkling of my humanness detectable in the document was flagged the way an English teacher circles misspelled words in red ink. A lemur kiss could only credibly be described as "lip-to-lip-contact," and I should not dare to assume that the intention of the lemur kisser has anything to do with love or affection. I understand and value that lesson as it pertains to the study of animal behavior, but now I proudly anthropomorphize. I believe it is inevitable. I also believe that the only people who have a real problem with anthropomorphism are those who are still attached to the dichotomy between humans and beyond-human beings. Do cats *felipomorphize* dogs? Probably, but I don't see scientists all in a tizzy about it!

The problem with anthropomorphism is that it enforces the boundary between us and other. Yes, anthropomorphism can be used superficially or to inappropriate ends. We must engage in it with a reflective mind, anthropomorphizing from a point of connection and curiosity instead of using it as a barrier that limits our understanding of our fellow animals. But we have no choice. The ways in which we perceive the world are human. Human animal. The fear of anthropomorphism and the distance it creates between individuals are far more harmful than the animal-to-animal connections inspired and initiated by it. Relating to other animals and seeking connections between our experience of the world and theirs is natural and often mutually beneficial, not to mention beautiful.

Some scientists have argued that it is a pointless waste of time to attempt to consider the world through the perspectives of other animals. Not surprisingly, I disagree. We must at least attempt this noble feat, if we are to avoid *anthropodenial,* a term coined by esteemed primatologist Frans de Waal.[2] Anthropodenial occurs when humans deny that beyond-human beings might share certain characteristics with us, or vice versa, when we deny that we are animals. And while we may never know what it is like to be a terrestrial snail snacking on mycelium, it is a mistake not to try to imagine the myriad earthy flavors as we chomp with thousands of mollusk choppers. To avoid anthropodenial, according to scholars such as Jane Bennett[3] and Radhika Govindrajan,[4] we need imagination, creativity, play, and attention to the senses. Human children, much like beaver kits, bear cubs, and gecko hatchlings, excel at this more easily than adults. This is where yoga comes in.

The word *yoga* comes from the Sanskrit for "to yoke, to unify, unite, connect."[5] There are eight limbs of yoga including *asana, pranayama* (breath regulation), *pratyahara* (withdrawal of the senses), *dharana* (concentration), *dhyana* (meditation), *yamas* (social ethics), *niyamas* (personal ethics), and *samadhi* (integrated union). Yoga is so much more than asana. Practice the poses, sure, but to understand yoga more deeply, I recommend exploring all eight limbs for yourself. Breathe with intention. Live an ethical life. Engage with and give back to your community. Read the yoga philosophy classics such as the *Bhagavad Gita* and *Autobiography of a Yogi,* study with experienced teachers, and decide what yoga practices resonate for you the most. Be who you are and feel what Stephen Cope calls the "warm animal of your body."[6]

I am not a yoga expert. I teach yoga, but I am a student first and foremost, always learning more. I am grateful to my teachers and my teachers' teachers' teachers all the way back to the origins of this tradition in South Asia. I know what yoga is to me, and I know that my yoga is different from that of the person next to me. This is the core message of this book. We are different, but we can share experiences with other beings that teach us, transform us, and convince us otherwise. Our forms may be different, but we are also all the same. All one, divine being. That is yoga. The union that occurs when we partner the movements of our body with our breath in our asana practice is an example, writ small, of what yoga means to me: union of our individual selves with the universal, divine Self.

The way yoga is practiced today is historically influenced by multiple Eastern religions, including Hinduism and Buddhism. Ancient yogis embodied this wisdom in every aspect of their lives, in contrast to yoga practitioners today who incorporate only certain aspects of the tradition into their modern, day-to-day routines. The level of commitment and intensity of practice is what distinguishes a yogi from a casual student who practices asana a couple of times a week and dabbles occasionally in the other seven limbs. Neither is "better" than the other, but it is a distinction worth mentioning. You do not have to agree with my definition of yoga, and you do not have to subscribe to any particular religion to practice asana, the physical component of yoga. According to *The Yoga Sutras of Patanjali,* one popular interpretation of yoga, asana is defined as a steady, comfortable posture, *sthira sukham,*[7] that was originally practiced to prepare the body for meditation.[8]

The original yogic texts, the Vedas, presented the first yoga teachings around 1500–1000 BCE. The texts include three human obligations, one of which, in the words of Maya Tiwari, is "reverence to the divine, reverence to nature—to the earth, river, wind, fire, and space, to the animals, plants, and every blade of grass, every speck of dust."[9] The *Gheranda Samhita*, a classic text on hatha yoga from the seventeenth century, also confirms the divine nature of nature: "All the creatures of the earth, all the creatures of the air, plants such as trees, shrubs, creepers, vines, grasses, water, and mountains: know all these to be Brahman and see them all in the self."[10] Brahman, in this context, refers to the universal, Ultimate Reality, or what I call oneness.

The *Gheranda Samhita* also suggests a direct link between animals and asana: "All together there are as many asanas as there are species of living beings."[11] While someone familiar with both yoga and biology understands that this number is always changing, the intriguing connection between the two reinforces the claim suggesting that there are as many versions of a pose as there are yoga practitioners because everyone's bodies and experiences are different. Historically, students were instructed to practice pranayama atop antelope or tiger skins,[12] and kundalini yoga *kriyas* are practiced on sheepskins. Today, plants and animals still support our asana practice quite literally in the form of yoga props like cork blocks, wool and cotton blankets, silk cushions filled with buckwheat hulls, and rubber mats.

Contemporary yoga teacher and advocate Susanna Barkataki reminds us that yoga originated "in an Indic culture that respected and learned from nature,"[13] so it makes sense for us to seek out props for our own practice that are made of natural materials. The last time I shopped for a new yoga mat I discovered Juru, a woman-founded, India-based company that makes yoga mats from naturally sourced cork and rubber. While not all my props are 100 percent natural, I consider it part of living my yoga to use sustainable and eco-friendly products whenever possible, and not to get caught up in unnecessary yoga industry consumerism. In fact, you can practice yoga without any specialized gear at all.

In the Hindu tradition, Lord Shiva, one of three central deities, is believed to have brought each animal into the world by practicing the asana that represents it, simultaneously creating both. When he first practiced *ustrasana,* for example, camels came into being. After practicing millions of poses, as many animals were created.[14] For this reason, Shiva is also sometimes known as Pashupati, protector of the animals. Additionally, some Hindus believe that humans must live as beyond-human beings 8,400,000 times, and are born through as many animal wombs.[15] The *Bhagavad Gita,* another Hindu scripture that details a conversation between a warrior (Arjuna) and God (Krishna), urges us to rejoice "in the welfare of all beings," and states that God loves best one "who treats all beings with kindness and compassion" because the Lord dwells equally in the hearts of all creatures.[16] Humans who achieve oneness know in their disposable bones that their self and every being is divine.

In Buddhism, the lives of people and animals are also interconnected. We share the same world and the same suffering.[17] Thus, the Boddhisatva vow contains a promise to lead all the universe's creatures from separation to unity, from misery to bliss. In the Mahayana tradition, people believe that humans have been reborn as every species, taking a variety of shapes and forms through countless reincarnations.[18] Perhaps we *can* know the experience of another animal after all. According to multiple religious traditions we have already known each one intimately.

Scrolls from the ninth-century Buddhist *Diamond Sutra* instruct that the notions of *human being, living being,* and *lifespan* prevent our liberation and keep us separate. Buddhist teacher Thich Nhat Hanh elaborates: "It's not only that we *were* a cloud or a rock in the past, but we *are* still a cloud and a rock today. In former times we were also a fish, a bird, a reptile."[19] We are in all things, and all things are in us. If a species goes extinct, we die with them because we are them. There is no finite lifespan because we are constantly changing and dying and being reborn. A lifespan works only within a conception of reality that includes linear time. In the same book, *Zen and the Art of Saving the Planet,* Buddhist nun Sister Chan Khong writes, "The seed of awakening and love is there in you and in all people and all species on Earth."[20]

If asana should be *sthira sukham,*[21] then nothing could be steadier or more comfortable than embodying earth's fellow creatures. I seek this experience of unity by exploring the space where animals and yoga overlap. Yes, many yoga poses are named after animals, and that is the starting point for this endeavor. But why are certain yoga poses named after certain animals, and what does this mean for individual students of yoga and our relationships with other beings? It suddenly becomes very strange that we practice something called "cobra pose" hundreds of times without thinking at all about the animal called a cobra as we do it. In *Eating Stone: Imagination and the Loss of the Wild,* Ellen Meloy wrote, "Shall we be honest about this? The mind needs wild animals. The body needs the trek that it takes looking for them."[22] While she referred to literal treks through the desert to observe bighorn sheep, I believe that asana is one of the ways our bodies can embark on a similar trek, resulting in an embodied connection to other animals and to wildness through yoga.

More than anything else, teaching nature yoga to kids has taught me that yoga is not something that happens on a 68 x 24-inch squishy mat made of synthetic materials. With children, we put our toes in the grass and yell 'til our voices echo in the surrounding hills. We wiggle and laugh and deny our humanness in pursuit of a more universal understanding. How does a coyote sing, a beaver stay warm in winter, or a snake move through the grass? The answers are endless, obvious, and effortless to children. They are found in the body. In *Coyote's Guide to Connecting with Nature,* authors Jon Young, Ellen Haas, and Evan McGown write: "The practice of imitating animal movement, which includes its mood and strategy, creates a meaningful relationship with the animal.... Playing with the forms of different animals teaches without words that each animal presents a unique and valid way of existing in the world.... We can have access to all these different perspectives on how to be alive."[23] Typically, when animals mimic each other, one is attempting to look or behave like another who has a certain survival advantage, such as poison or aggression, that protects them from predation.[24] While yoga asana doesn't help most of us to survive in a direct, day-to-day kind of way, there is no doubt that yoga and its associated practices, including the mimicking of other animals, improve the mental and physical health of regular practitioners,[25] making it a little easier to survive after all.

If yoga practitioners seek to understand the world, in part, through immediate experience,[26] then we should also seek to learn about other beings before imitating them with our bodies. This doesn't mean we cannot practice scorpion pose without first seeing a scorpion. There are books and poems and pictures and videos and stories—many ways of experiencing other animals without being in their immediate physical presence. There are people who research elusive animals, such as critically endangered snow leopards, who study their whole lives without ever laying eyes on one. There is so much about other beings we don't now (and may never) know. But there is much more to learn from what our own experiences and senses can teach us. Then we can attempt to become animal in mind, to explore what those connections feel like in the body. Yet you don't have to behave like one to be one. People with limited mobility or other varying abilities can embody these animals and connect with them through various forms of mindful movement and thought. Yoga is for everyone. So is connecting with nature.

This advice to embody beyond-human beings through mimicry and play is not reserved for children, but the older we get the more challenging it becomes. The circles *play* and *yoga* in the Venn diagram of life overlap in childhood but grow farther apart as we age. Yoga for adults is rarely promoted as fun—it is for our physical and mental health, our mobility, our self-care, our ability to function in society with comfort and ease. We forget that the true goal of yoga is Yoga—union—with the divine, which includes beyond-human beings. The not-so-fun underlying assumption here is that we are currently separated. From other humans, certainly from other animals, and even from ourselves. This is the root problem.

As many yoga practitioners know, barriers to understanding others and achieving oneness are often created and perpetuated by our own minds. What a strange problem! We are not actually separate; we merely perceive that we are. If we achieve true yoga, there is no distinction between human, animal, or the divine, and the journey toward this unity can be playful. We can be outside in the fresh air, watching other animals and meditating on the marvels of their lives. We can practice yoga in view of bird feeders or on hiking trails, while howling at a starry sky or paddling down a spring-fed river.

So *how* do we become animal on the yoga mat? When we go in search of connection with other beings, we forget that we *are* that which we seek.[27] Identifying as human creates separation. Embodying animals through yoga teaches us that not only are we more same than different but also that we are all *the same*. As Susanna Barkataki wrote, "Yoga supports us with tools, a framework and practices to undo separation and create equity and unity."[28] Yoga helps us break down the unproductive dichotomy between human and animal that pervades our society. Luckily, modern studies in neuroscience, cognition, and ethology—the study of animal behavior—make it increasingly difficult to cling to this dualistic point of view.[29]

Practicing yoga (or any mindful or devotional practice) outside like the early yogis, for example, can help us to feel more connected. Then, we are more likely to act with compassion toward all living beings, both on and off our yoga mats. If we want to feel fresh air in our bodies, why not go outside where there are no barriers between oxygen-producing trees and our noses, between carbon-dioxide-thirsty trees and our mindful exhales? If we want to experience clarity of mind, why not go outside where there are no walls to trap our suffering and no ceilings to impede our view of the seemingly infinite sky? If we want to feel one with other beings, why not practice in their homes and their habitats only to recall what we have always known— that their homes and habitats are, of course, also our own? Micah Mortali wrote that praying outside "allows the more-than-human world to interact with me in moments of vulnerable conversation with the mystery of life."[30] When we connect our bodies and our breath to nature, we are more likely to feel a sense of oneness, to experience union.

Wild asana is the antidote to anthropodenial and an invitation to anthropomorphize with abandon. It can help to treat "species loneliness"[31] and to guide us on the journey of "rewilding our hearts."[32] I hope this book helps you not to become animal only for a moment as you explore a certain pose, but to realize that you have truly and always been animal. You breathe and move with intention. You use your senses to remember the present over and over again. Your body knows what you need.

There are thirteen chapters in this book. Included are essays about five mammals, three reptiles, two birds, a fish, an insect, and an arachnid. There is a corpse at the end. And a mountain. Chapters can be read out of order if you feel drawn to explore a certain creature, but they are also organized in such a way that reading the book straight through follows a logical flow. In each one, I write about my own observations in nature and how our yoga practice can connect us to beyond-human beings, but the asana is really just a tool. A skill that moves us into action.[33] If connection is the nail and yoga is the hammer, then our ultimate goal is neither. It is beyond connection. Our goal is the metal that composes both the hammer and the nail. Beyond connection is becoming one being. Embodiment, unity. Yoga with a capital Y. It is no easy task, but the practices included at the end of each chapter are designed to inspire your journey. Even if you don't practice them, you may begin to think about how to apply the concepts from my own quirky animal brain, and all the wise beings I have cited, into your own life.

I am not enlightened or one with anything, but I do know that I have caught little glimmers of oneness during my experiences in connection with beyond-human beings and with nature . . . in the glimpse of the cottontail's white pouf disappearing into the brush, in the whisper of the woodcock foraging in the shrubland, and in the whiff of my dog after we play in the rain. Connecting with beyond-human beings through a practice as intimate, in-the-body, and transformative as yoga, brings us an arm's, a wing's, a fin's length closer to union.

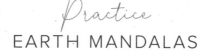

EARTH MANDALAS

Mandala is the Sanskrit word for "circle." Mandalas are used in many of the world's cultures and religions as devotional images with geometric patterns that symbolize the universe in its ideal form. The creation of a mandala is a sacred practice that signifies the transformation of the universe from suffering to joy. Examples of mandalas in nature include flowers, eyeballs, tree rings, snowflakes, spiderwebs, shells, fruits, and more. Creating nature mandalas can help us to:

- Remember and honor our connection to the earth
- Express gratitude
- Slow down and cultivate mindful attention

- Acknowledge the cyclical and continuous nature of life
- Observe and enjoy patterns found in nature
- Appreciate the little, often-overlooked things
- Express our creativity
- Practice nonattachment and impermanence
- Have fun!

To make an earth mandala, choose a peaceful place in nature. Prepare the surface by clearing debris and sprinkling water to symbolically purify the spot, or reflecting on your intention to create. Gather organic materials (twigs, leaves, grasses, flowers, berries, pinecones, acorns, etc.). Of course, be aware of your surroundings. Watch out for poison oak or ivy and try not to disturb critters. Take only the materials you will use. Place a single meaningful item in the center and assemble the other materials in a symmetrical pattern around it. Consider color, texture, size, and shape as you arrange the items. When you are finished, take a few moments to appreciate your mandala. Finally, destroy or abandon it. It is meant to be temporary. Let go, and let nature take over your creation.

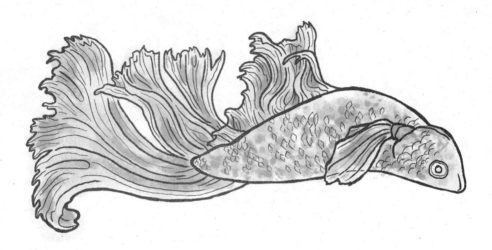

Chapter 1

MATSYA—FISH

I am an earth gal. A Virgo. A researcher of and advocate for terrestrial creatures (okay, some admittedly arboreal, and some semiaquatic), I am most comfortable with my two feet firmly planted on the earth's surface. While dogs, cats, corvids, and babies understand the concept of object permanence, I doubt it myself when I can no longer see the ground from any air or water vessel. If I am out on the water, I prefer to be able to see the shore. If I am underground, I better be able to sense the sunshine at the surface. When I fly, I am least anxious looking down at the solid earth. Plane rides, tunnels, caves, coal mines, and the open ocean scare me. And although I still have the Certificate of Achievement that I earned after completing my swimming lessons in the early nineties like a dutiful Floridian, the most salient memory I have of that experience is of the river rock gravel that covered the pool deck in shades of red and brown, whose rough and uneven texture comforted my pruney feet at the end of each class.

Despite my connection to earth instead of water, I was baptized at Temple Terrace Community Church on Sunday, December 25, in the "year of our Lord" 1988. After a live solo of "Ave Maria," the beloved family minister took me into his arms and sprinkled holy water on my head, taking care to tilt me backward so the water didn't trickle into my face.

"You were real good!" my mom recalled.

I didn't cry or fuss like some babies do, but in a photograph from that day, I looked unenthused, as I suppose a three-month-old in a fancy knit dress with wet wisps of hair should feel. Truthfully, it is how I still feel about my baptism: ambivalent and mostly unattached to its significance. At least there was a poinsettia in honor of my christening that day, rooted firmly in a pot of dirt, to balance out the earth baby on her damp first Christmas.

"It was assumed back then that babies would get baptized. Not a great deal of thought went into it," my mom explained. "We just wanted you to be exposed to something."

My parents were baptized in Protestant churches to which their families weren't terribly attached. They attended services on Christmas and Easter and sporadically in between, finding comfort in the community but lacking conviction in the associated dogma. Honestly, my relationship with Christianity isn't nearly as fraught as that of many of my friends who, as adults, have grappled with their parents' faith and reckoned with its less-than-holy influence on their ideas of gender roles, marriage equality, and other human rights issues.

Babies, adults, and all ages in between across the Christian world are sprinkled, doused, or dunked in water because John the Baptist did so to Jesus. In some churches there is a heated baptismal pool and in others a small bowl. Some congregations head down to the nearest creek. Nevertheless, the action symbolizes a rebirth, a religious cleansing, and the forgiveness of sins.[1] In the book of Mark, which was originally written in Greek, baptisms not only occurred in the river; they occurred *into* the river. Pastor and biblical scholar Victoria Loorz points out the relational nature of the Greek word *eis*, or "into," which is often translated as "in" in English. The baptism did not simply occur at the arbitrary location of the River Jordan. The river herself was part of it. Jesus was not baptized in the River Jordan; he was baptized into union with her. Into meaningful relationship with the living, wild waters, with God, and with nature. Among aquatic plants and wildlife like Mesopotamian barb fishes who fed on the river bottom[2] while mud and pebbles squelched between Jesus's toes. Loorz wrote, "Baptism into a river is a wilderness immersion that initiates an intimate, vulnerable union with the living world."[3]

If we consider baptism in those terms, the day I was *really* baptized was sometime in 2003, on an overnight school trip to the MarineLab science education center in Key Largo. One morning, we took a short boat ride to a coral reef to snorkel. At some point, floating in the water with oversized flippers jostling on my feet behind me, I was enveloped into a school of blue fishes. For that one ethereal moment there was nothing in the world but blue fishes—above me, below me, and inches from my body in every direction. I was immersed into them, swallowed by them in the best possible way (not like the "Jonah is in trouble with God" kind of way). These fishes were beautiful. They were the solid shade of my all-time favorite Crayola crayon—cerulean—with neon-lined crescent moon tails, puckered lips, and expressive eyeballs that you could only see one at a time. Confident in their monochromatism, they had no need for flashy crisp lines or complementary-colored fins. They were made for the water, all body bulk and very little fin, with a subtle pattern that resembled the foam trail left behind from waves lapping on a sandy shore.

It lasted only a few seconds. In the middle of that school of fishes I forgot all that a fourteen-year-old girl worries about: the fit of my bathing suit and the shape and size of my body within it, whether my crush was nearby, and whom I was going to sit with in the cafeteria for dinner. I remember popping upright in the water after the fishes moved on and spitting out my rubber mouthpiece to verify with my snorkel buddy that what we experienced was not a dream. I certainly didn't have the words to describe the experience then, but I knew that when I emerged from that salty water and peeled off my wetsuit, I had a new sense of awe for the world.

On that same trip we observed bioluminescent plankton lighting up the night sea, pufferfishes camouflaged and unpuffed, intimidating teeth protruding from the mouths of barracudas as long as our bodies, and pop-eyed parrotfishes foraging for algae among the coral. But nothing beat my momentary membership in a school of Atlantic blue tang. I was baptized into nature, into the sea off the southern coast of my home state, and into new relationship with beyond-human beings who once felt foreign but were now part of me forever. I was a wide-eyed, slightly salty, teenage fish mystic; I just didn't know it yet. Perhaps my baptism-as-baby in the church sanctuary lacked meaning because I was not immersed into the water among the beings who call it home. Surely the gentle waves of the Atlantic Ocean are as holy as the water dripping from the minister's fingers.

In the classroom at MarineLab we learned that the Atlantic blue tang was in the surgeonfish family. I recall giggling with my friends at the term *caudal peduncle*, which refers to the tapered part of the fish, in front of the tail, where blue tangs have sharp spines that they use to defend themselves. They are constantly munching on algae and cleaning other fishes and sea turtles in a mutual interspecies exchange of services in their bustling reef communities. When they need cleaning, they perform headstands for little gobies who remove parasites from their bodies. Clean and be cleaned—just another version of baptism on the reef!

Clearly, the blue tangs I had the pleasure of meeting that day were in schooling mode, traveling in a large group so they could move faster, forage more effectively, and benefit from increased protection from predators. Fishes who school are masters at tuning into the movements of others, of paying attention to nuances of being beyond our human capability. They can sense each other's movements with such accuracy because of an organ called the lateral line, a collection of special scales that function like sonar and allow them to move in sync as if one giant fish, or at least, a lot of individual fishes with one mind. Indeed, the social lives of fishes are quite complex. They recognize each other as individuals,[4] enjoy each other's touch,[5] and engage in consensus decision-making.[6] They learn from each other and engage in social play, sometimes with other species, including humans. Many reef fishes have such intricate intra- and interspecies relationships that it is not far-fetched at all to claim that they have culture.[7] Knowing this, I especially cannot believe that those blue tangs decided to make me a part of their group, even for a moment, that day.

I remember when I used to believe that fishes had poor memories. I thought that was what made them mindful. It's easy to stay in the present when the past was three seconds ago. Yet multiple studies have proved that fishes have great memories. One research project inadvertently discovered that goldfishes have memories lasting a year or longer when they relate to the color and location of a food source.[8] And gobies can memorize tide pools at high tide so they can jump from one to the other at low tide in an impressive display of both memory and cognitive mapping skills.[9]

❋ ❋ ❋

I grew up with a little hexagonal fish tank of rotating residents and the emotional immunity that results from routinely flushing the small bodies of your pets down the toilet (something my husband first heard about in his thirties with a little shock and not a little judgment). That is not to say that I didn't love my finned friends. In elementary school, I was assigned an essay about my hero, and I chose to write about my pet fish, a zebra danio named— wait for it—Danny. Admittedly, the most impressive thing about him in my memory was the fact that he outlived all his tank-mates. When I moved into my college dorm room and couldn't stand the thought of life without pets, I bought two guppies and named them Jim and Dwight after characters from *The Office*, but I never did have luck with guppies . . . flush, flush. Later, I got a betta fish named Siddhartha, Sid for short. The fish buddha.

According to the Jatakas, the collection of stories from the Buddha's former incarnations, the Buddha himself spent at least one lifetime help- ing other fishes avoid suffering and attain happiness by freeing them from fishermen's nets and causing heavy rains in response to life-threatening droughts. According to the *Aryasura Jatakas*, "The Great Being felt as ten- derly toward those fish, as if they were his own beloved offspring, and in various ways he showed them great kindness."[10] We have strayed greatly from this perspective.

In the aquarium trade, fishes are often treated as objects instead of com- panions, kept largely for their beauty and ornamental appeal.[11] It is why we find betta fishes swimming—no, slumping—in tiny cups of cloudy water in cubbies at the pet store. I used to strain to avert my eyes from this depress- ing sight every time I bought dog food. Then one day I decided, "Not this time," and I bought one. A blue, iridescent, shimmery specimen whose cup said "Male Butterfly," but whose color said, "Like my blue tang school- mates of faraway waters."

I am fully aware that buying a betta in a cup at a pet store conglomerate supports the system that puts the fishes in the cups to begin with. I did not "rescue" this fish, but I did purchase for him a new tank, a low-flow filter, a water heater, a variety of live plants, a floating hollow log, and a leaf hammock on which to slumber. Poor Siddhartha lived in a glass bowl of room-temperature water for years, but I did my research this time. It is our responsibility to treat all pets, whether Great Danes or guppies, with love and respect to the best of our abilities, and to ensure that they live happy, healthy lives and die dignified deaths. No more flushes here. We're a fish-burying household now!

I named my new gilled companion Matsya, the Sanskrit word for fish,[12] and set up his aquarium in my home office. He keeps me company as I write. In my attempt to care for Matsya as best as I possibly can, I read books about betta-keeping and joined online groups of betta fanatics. Sadly, none of these resources answered my most pressing questions. I don't need a whole chapter on how to breed an award-winning steel blue half-moon veil tail. I want to know if Matsya can hear me speaking to him and if he can recognize my voice, and what do voices sound like to him through the glass and the water, and his internal fish versions of ears. What does it feel like to live in that flowy, finny body? What do fishes think? What do they hate? Whom do they love?

From books I did learn many fascinating things about fishes and how they exist in their watery world. They use tools, for example. Some species crack open shellfish with rocks and some carry around eggs glued to a leaf.[13] They cooperate with others in their school and with other species to hunt, find food, clean, and be cleaned.[14] Many fishes can plan ahead and engage in complex thinking.[15] Archerfishes from Asia and Australia shoot powerful streams of water from their mouths to knock bugs from mangrove branches into the water to eat. While hunting, these fishes assess the size and type of prey before choosing the amount of water and style of shooting needed for optimum success.[16] Koi have learned to distinguish between different musical genres and goldfishes can be trained to identify shapes.[17] Some fishes can identify themselves in a mirror.[18] Some fishes create art. Male white-spotted pufferfishes make mandalas in the sand and decorate the grooves with shells to attract a mate.[19] (The fact that there is a natural phenomenon for which I can use the words *pufferfish* and *mandala* in the same sentence brings me great joy.)

About bettas specifically, I read that their Latin name, *Betta splendens*, means "splendid warrior," after an ancient Malay warrior tribe. Others call them Siamese fighting fish, and indeed, betta fishes were domesticated for fighting competitions. Now they are bred, kept, and sold all over the world. Their wild counterparts live in wet rice paddies,[20] known in Indonesia as *sawah,* that resemble endless layers of green framed with banana leaves, somehow ordered and chaotic at the same time. The scenery is equally stunning on a clear, sunny day or a gloomy and gray one, shrouded in mist. Up close they look like steps but from afar they undulate like waves. It is no surprise that some of the most beautiful fishes I've ever seen have been bred from a species that inhabits one of the most beautiful landscapes I've ever seen.

I've become interested in creating an environment that mimics what Matsya's habitat would be like in the wild. His tank is long and relatively shallow because bettas prefer to swim side-to-side with easy access to the water's surface (I can relate), from which they gulp air with their labyrinthine organs. If Matsya had a mate, he would use this skill to build a nest, a collection of floating bubbles, to protect his eggs. Live plants offer hiding spots and natural water-purifying capabilities. I float an Indian almond leaf in the tank to add tannins that darken the water, lower its pH, and provide antibacterial and antifungal benefits. Fishes have lots of taste buds,[21] so I feed Matsya floating pellets that come in a variety of flavors, and occasionally, worms (frozen, then thawed) to mimic a more natural diet of opportunistically caught critters. He relishes the blood worms I squirt into the water with a pipette, as they appear to swim for a split second before he hunts and slurps their crimson bodies like noodles in soup. Bettas also sleep near the water's surface. When I spied Matsya on the first night I brought him home, he was sleeping in the little leaf hammock that I suction-cupped to the glass.

As I write this, I look toward the tank and wonder if Matsya is playing hide-and-seek with me. He seems to sense me looking and swims back and forth in the corner closest to my desk before darting behind a leaf. The way his blue fins billow is otherworldly. Bettas are truly the puppy dogs of the freshwater aquarium world. After reading that some captive fishes enjoy human touch,[22] I decide to put this idea to the test. I unplug the tank's heater and reach my (clean) hand into the seventy-eight-degree water. Matsya swims in circles around me, cautious yet curious, but does not touch my hand.

Some people suggest that encouraging males to flare by showing them a mirror is a healthy form of exercise and enrichment in moderation. The first time I put a mirror in front of Matsya, he didn't react. Now that he is well settled in his new home, he spreads his expanse of fins and flares at the mirror that I float in his tank for a couple of minutes every few days. I also notice, with satisfaction, that his colors have deepened and darkened since he came to live with me. (The online betta folks call this a "glow-up.") The awe I experience watching Matsya echoes the feeling I had when I was baptized with the blue tangs all those years ago. I touch my puckered lips to the glass and wonder what he thinks of the goofy human face in front of his own.

Fishes are often talked about and interacted with as though they are commodities rather than individuals. As Jonathan Balcombe writes in *What a Fish Knows*, "If there is one overarching conclusion we can draw from the current science on fishes, it is this: fishes are not merely alive—they have lives."[23] Language can either strengthen and inspire our relationships with nature or obscure them altogether. Use of the term *fish* as both singular and plural robs these animals of agency and denies the existence of single, individual fishes.[24] Even the verb *to fish* takes away the very fish-ness—the essence—of the animals and removes them from the environment in which they became fishes in the first place.

Our interactions with fishes are also characterized by consumption. From fishing-for-fun to the large-scale fishing-for-food industry, the intrinsic value of these animals is degraded with every reference to stock, catch, and harvest. Those two fishes that Jesus used to feed thousands of people in John 6:1–14 were both separate beings with personalities and individual experiences of the world.

In Makassar, Indonesia, I used to frequent a specific restaurant to eat *ikan laut*, ocean fish. When my friends and I walked in, the host opened a cooler and we pointed to the freshly caught fishes we wanted to eat.

"Dibakar atau digoreng?" the man asked. Grilled or fried?

There was no wrong choice—it was all delicious, especially with a generous squeeze of lime and our go-to side dish of *kangkung*, sauteed water spinach with copious amounts of garlic, and thirst-quenching Bintang beer. Depending on the fish and preparation method we chose, some-times it came to the table prepared whole and sometimes flayed open. We picked around the bones and eyeballs with only slight hesitation and waited weeks in between visits to the city for more delicious *ikan laut*. Would I have been as eager to eat the fresh kill of the day instead of the fresh catch?

Years later my husband and I spent the morning *ooh*ing and *aah*ing at fishes at the National Aquarium in Baltimore and then beelined it to the nearest seafood restaurant at the harbor for lunch. The irony was not lost on me that day, and it continues to both amuse and disturb me, although I did eventually stop eating fishes. Then I stumbled upon a quote from Ingrid Newkirk that perfectly sums up our hypocrisy: "Killing fishes who you don't know is just part of the culture."[25] To human beings, fishes are food, beloved pet, decoration, and recreation. What contradictions these beyond-human beings so unlike our own bodies embody!

Fishes are symbols of freedom[26] and enlightenment[27] in Buddhism, yet they are supposedly incapable of feeling pain. *Do* fishes feel pain? For a long time, humans have questioned this idea simply because fishes don't express themselves the ways that we do.[28] This is when anthropomorphism gets us into trouble. If fishes' eyes don't blink, or cry, or squeeze shut in a wince, we assume they don't feel pain. But if projecting our humanness onto animals also means that when they don't behave like we do, we assume they don't feel anything, then that's a problem! If we think other animals should react the same way to a stimulus that we do in order to believe that response is valid, then anthropomorphism has led us astray.

There is scientific evidence that fishes feel both the sharp initial pains and the long-lasting aches that follow bodily injury. Although some human anglers report different experiences, fishes remember places where they felt pain and subsequently avoid those places.[29] We have a cerebral cortex and fishes do not;[30] but just because our brains look different doesn't imply that one of us feels pain and the other doesn't. I hope our brains look differ-ent! There are millions of years of ongoing evolution separating us, but that doesn't mean that feeling pain doesn't also help fishes to avoid dangerous situations. We all want to survive.

Fishes feel emotional pain, too. They react physiologically to stress like we do, with increased adrenaline and cortisol production. Stress in fishes can be fatal in captive scenarios when territorial disputes play out in cramped conditions and a single individual is confined to a corner of the tank without access to food and social interaction.[31] When captive fishes are depressed (housed alone in tanks with little enrichment) they respond positively to drugs used to treat mental illness in humans.[32] Even if fishes didn't feel pain, it doesn't seem to justify hooks through lips, suffocation in trawling nets, and lives in barren bowls. Survival is not enough. We all also want to thrive. What if we treated fishes as if they could feel pain, whether we believe they do or not? We could show them respect and compassion, regardless of what semantic labels we feel the need to impose on our fellow beings.

※ ※ ※

If Matsya is fish, then matsyasana is fish pose. It is one of my favorite asanas despite its status as a heart-opener, a pose that requires intense expansion of the chest. I don't typically enjoy heart-opening poses because of the physical and emotional vulnerability they require. I can never tell if it is the shape of my body or the state of my mind that makes breathing in the pose difficult. Matsyasana begins from a supine position, lying on the ground on the back, face up. I place my hands underneath my bottom as my chest and shoulders start to open. Then, in a complex sequence of simultaneous movement, three things occur at once: lifting my heart, pressing weight into my forearms, and touching the crown of my head to the ground. I flare my gills like a territorial betta fish, a little belligerent about it. Matsyasana feels like that fish on my plate in Makassar: flayed open, but instead of dead and cooked, very alive.

I embrace the strength of my form as scales slowly cover my body. Two legs become one because fishes don't have such things. With toes (what are those?) angled and askew, there is no question that my feet are no longer feet, but a fish tail, and my ankles a damn fine caudal peduncle—with sharp spine or without? It depends on my mood. If I stay in matsyasana long enough, the air around me turns to water. For a split-second I fear drowning, but then I remember my gills. I am not a commodity. I am different from the fish next to me, who is immersed in the waters of her own experience.

We are individuals; yet, we are linked together like a school, tuned into the watery world around us, lateral lines ablaze, open to encounters with others and moving, immersed in infinite waves of change.

Many creatures obtain their oxygen with organs and strategies entirely different from our own. I've had occasional and relatively mild panic attacks since before I knew what they were, since before I spent a single full decade on the earth in this body. They got worse in my twenties and often happened when I was driving alone at night. I remember telling my dad (and retired psychiatrist) that no matter how much deep, yogic breathing I tried, the frantic feelings only seemed to worsen. His matter-of-fact reply changed everything.

"Your deep breathing is fueling the panic with more oxygen. Try holding your breath instead."

I had been blowing on the fire. This simple trick of breathing less instead of more worked wonders for managing my panic attacks, but it also changed the way I think about pranayama, the yogic practice of breath control and another of yoga's eight limbs. While there are certainly benefits to a pranayama practice, I am convinced that we tend to overthink it. It is very human of us to manipulate the breath for purposes beyond breathing (and communicating, which some other animals do too). Other beings don't consciously micromanage their breath like we do. We forget that our animal bodies know how to breathe whether our minds are involved or not. Breath is both simpler and far more complex than it seems. It is also *prana*, the life force that is shared with all beings, connecting us to others in an inevitable exchange of oxygen and much more.

Embodying a fish may seem like a special stretch of the imagination because we are so physically different—our primate selves and these little aliens we call fishes. Matsya lives in water; I live on land. Matsya uses his nostrils only for smelling, while mine also help me breathe. Matsya has a tail, and I have feet. Yet, fishes are more like us than we think. Truthfully, I resent the fact that I need to argue that. I cringe at the assumption that to take other animals and their well-being seriously we need to compare instead of contrast them with our own also-animal selves. I believe we can let the gilled and finned into our hearts as gracefully as we open our chests in fish pose— not despite, but because of, those differences. If we all had the same body types or experiences, these yoga poses would be us just standing around like bipedal ape doofuses!

It is one thing to study and understand how fishes experience the world, but matsyasana requires that we become the fish. Even this is possible. If we reflect on our own experiences in water and how it alters our senses, being fish is suddenly more accessible. Underwater our sight is blurred, our hearing amplified yet distorted, our sense of gravity and movement transformed. In the bathtub or the swimming pool we can reconnect to these sensations. The sensitivity to the temperature of the water on our skin, our hairs floating away from our skull and waving like fins. Buoyant peace. Immersion into divine waters. This is what it's like to be matsya.

After all, the beginnings of this body were fish-like: a fetus suspended in amniotic fluid, a being beyond human. We breathed via umbilical cords until our lungs developed and we took our first real breaths at birth. In fact, our lungs evolved from swim bladders, sac-like organs filled with gas that fishes use to control their buoyancy.[33] Water isn't as foreign as my earth-loving self feared. I knew it in the womb and on Christmas day in 1988. The blue tangs and I, we both knew it years ago in the salty ocean, and Matsya and I, we both know it now. Water. We are made of the stuff, not separate from it. Just like the fishes.

Practice

BREATH RETENTION

You don't need to breathe like a fish or keep an aquarium to connect with a fish. Become a fish. Baptize yourself into nature. Visit a pond, a puddle, a spring, a river, an ocean. Acknowledge the fishes and other beyond-human beings who live there. You don't need anyone's blessing. The water falling from the sky and rushing down the hillside is already holy.

Get yourself in some water, the element that connects us to the fishes, the one thing we all need to survive and thrive. A bathtub, a pool, a bucket, or a bowl will do. Dip your hand in the water. If it is safe to do so, submerge ears, eyes, nose, and mouth. Hear like a fish and listen to sounds moving through the water. See underwater sights. Taste underwater flavors. Notice the water on your skin. What does it feel like? If the water is potable, take a sip and feel the liquid traveling down your esophagus. Open your heart and immerse yourself into knowing.

Hold your breath. The concept of *breath retention* in pranayama is called *kumbhaka*. It is a relatively advanced practice, best learned from an experienced teacher. Still, we've all held our breath for one reason or another—in fear or in awe, to become especially still or silent. The idea of conscious breath retention is meant to temporarily still the fluctuations of the mind. For advanced practitioners, breathing does not cease during kumbhaka; it continues in a more subtle way, like the difference between the ways that humans and fishes breathe oxygen. Pranayama teacher Richard Rosen suggests that when we practice breath retention, "We become more like our authentic self, still and serene, self-contained, joyful."[34]

To experiment with breath retention after the inhale (*antar-kumbhaka*), sit comfortably in a chair or on the floor. Inhale for six counts. (Note: A count does not equal a second. You choose the pace of your breath.) Exhale for six counts. Repeat until the pace of your breathing feels right. Then, at the end of an inhale, hold the breath for three counts. Don't tense up your body or grasp at your held breath. Simply pause. Exhale, and practice a few more rounds, taking three normal six-count breaths in between each retention.[35] It may help to consider how antar-kumbhaka allows you to savor the prana, to take advantage of the benefits of the air and energy in your lungs. Be especially mindful of this practice's effect on your state of mind. Take a brief break from breath, knowing that you will inhale again as soon as you need it. See if the practice calms and invigorates you. If it doesn't, stop and return to your natural breathing.

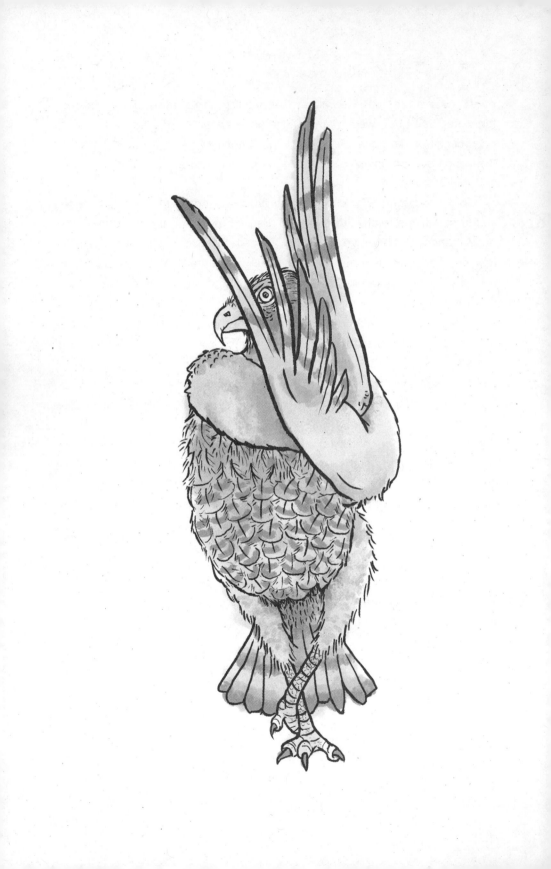

Chapter 2
GARUDA—EAGLE

Do eagles struggle with infertility? They used to. In Rachel Carson's *Silent Spring* we learned that on the west coast of Florida in the late 1940s, a researcher named Charles Broley observed a severe decline in the population of young bald eagles. A few years later, at Hawk Mountain in Pennsylvania, Maurice Brown observed the same trend—many more adult birds than juveniles migrating over this famous geographic bottleneck. Locations around the country reported similar results. Although eagles were nesting and laying eggs, eaglets were increasingly rare. Carson wrote that it was likely insecticide use that affected eagle reproduction, and subsequent studies confirmed it. Research on quail and pheasants revealed that the chemical compound nicknamed DDT (dichloro-diphenyl-trichloroethane) harmed the processes of egg production and embryo development and decreased hatchling survival rates. Traces of the insecticide were found in the reproductive organs of parent birds, eggs, embryos, and nestlings.[1]

I also struggle with infertility. Month after month, I pee on a stick and there is only one line. Not pregnant. It doesn't matter how many giant, stinking vitamins I swallow, how many cruciferous vegetables I eat, or how many needles the acupuncturist pokes into tender ankles and ears. It doesn't matter if I finish crocheting the baby blanket or not. The universe doesn't give a fuck that with a tangled ball of yarn and some woo-woo intention I think I am "ready" to get pregnant.

My husband and I endure the same routine every month, expecting different results. We "mate" as a scientist would say, in a scheduled, high-pressure kind of way during my alleged "fertile window"; then we wait and hope. One month I hoped because I had the HSG test, the one that is supposed to flush out your uterus and Fallopian tubes and increase the chance of conceiving. It didn't. Another couple of months I hoped because I was taking Clomid, a medicine to make me "super-ovulate." It gave me a migraine and blinding rage, but it didn't work. Even when I started to experience the telltale signs of PMS there was still hope, because every article I've ever Googled at 2:00 a.m. says that early pregnancy symptoms mimic the symptoms of PMS. Then I would take the high-stakes pee test, it would be negative, and my world would shatter again. And again. And again. Every month, without fail.

Do eagles know hope? Today, if an eagle lays eggs that never hatch, how does her avian heart bear it? For my human heart, this sorrow is not sustainable. At least infertile eagles don't have other well-meaning eagles saying things like, "You're still young and healthy," and "Just relax and have fun with it!" At least they don't have to attend eaglet showers and watch their friends open adorable onesies and tiny pairs of shoes. (Okay, for a second of some levity, imagine an eagle version of a onesie....) But eagles also don't have support groups like the lovely people I've met through mutual friends enduring similar experiences. Talking to others struggling with infertility is often the only thing that helps me feel truly understood. I hope that eagles, too, have some source of comfort in the event of an unexpectedly empty nest. An effortless fish catch on a cool, sunny day. Or an especially lengthy thermal of warm air for optimal soaring. A caring mate with which to share an evening roost, and the perfectly shaped branch for cozy slumber. For lucky eagles and privileged humans, there is assisted reproductive technology in the form of captive breeding efforts to conserve endangered raptors and in vitro fertilization.

✳ ✳ ✳

I used to think hope was something positive to motivate and inspire us in a world full of stress and heartbreak. Now, I understand that hope is not always a good thing. Sometimes it tortures us, taking us out of the present moment and causing suffering. Hope has us focusing on the future instead of right now, making us less mindful. Hoping for pregnancy feels like how I imagine those rescued eagles at the zoo feel, stuck on a perch but looking toward the sky. Instead, I try to embrace the teachings of Buddhist nun

Pema Chödrön, who advises us to "abandon hope" because "if we totally experience hopelessness, giving up all hope of alternatives to the present moment, we can have a joyful relationship with our lives."[2] Giving up hope alleviates suffering as we surrender to what is happening right now.

You may be concerned by the ease with which I trash the idea of hope in a chapter about reproducing to contribute to the next generation. Of course, my partner and I have questioned this whole endeavor. In the face of human-caused climate change and its increasingly severe effects, we wondered: Should we bring a child into this warming world? In the midst of a global pandemic, we wondered: Should we bring a child into this diseased world? When certain states proposed new legislation that discriminated against LGBTQ+ youth, we wondered: Should we bring a child into this intolerant world? As news of yet another mass shooting broke, this one targeting Black people shopping for groceries, we wondered: Should we bring a child into this racist, violent world? And when the Supreme Court overturned *Roe v. Wade*, we wondered: Should we bring a child into this misogynistic world? I even wondered about the concept of *biological carrying capacity* and nonbreeding due to high population density and low food availability. Could this idea apply to humans as it does to other animals like Eurasian beavers?[3] Does my body sense that the world is too dangerous or too crowded a place for raising young? Does it know that the world is a mess, so it shuts down attempts at reproduction?

Then I realized that if eagle mamas didn't continue sitting on those fragile eggs, DDT would have won. If we don't continue trying to conceive despite the current state of our world, then the fear and anxiety of an uncertain future wins. I believe that whether we incubate an embryo inside our own body, someone else's body, or under a brood patch devoid of feathers, when we bring new life into the world and raise our chicks and children with concern for others and the planet, collectively, we all win.

✳ ✳ ✳

"The way of the mystic is the way of surrender," wrote Mirabai Starr.[4] Do raptors know surrender? I've often wondered what eagle mamas felt when they sat on eggs that cracked and collapsed beneath their weight because of their unintentional ingestion of DDT. Not only did the chemical cause shell-thinning, but birds also exhibited behavioral problems caused by damage to their central nervous systems, and marine mammals such as sea lions gave birth to more premature and stillborn fetuses.[5] How many times did an individual animal experience such loss, and what were the effects on those who experienced it?

We know that other animals grieve. Anecdotal observations and scientific studies suggest that beyond-human beings from cows to corvids (i.e., crows and jays) to cetaceans (i.e., dolphins and whales) react to the passing of those with whom they lived and bonded, and even those who are stillborn. There are examples of dead infants groomed and carried by their primate mothers as the bodies decomposed, and dolphins who spent days guiding corpses of their calves to the surface to breathe while neglecting to feed themselves.[6]

While the experience of grief may differ for eagles, they must be in some way confused by broken eggshells or chicks cold and still, not begging for food. An eagle pair spends months building a large nest that they use year after year. I used to teach about the size of eagles' nests by having young students lie on the ground in a circle with their feet in the center to show nest width. Then they'd raise their arms to demonstrate depth. A female bald eagle lays up to three eggs per clutch and only one brood per year.[7] After nesting with such intention and incubating the precious few eggs for a month or more, certainly they expect their young to hatch and survive. Certainly, they feel something if they don't. Grief is not reserved for human beings.

Thankfully, DDT was banned in 1972, after which the Endangered Species Act provided federal protection for bald eagles in most states. Populations recovered over time. In 2001, the species' conservation status was changed from endangered to threatened.[8] Birders could once again watch in awe as juvenile eagles joined the flocks of raptors migrating across the country. And mated eagle pairs in Florida, Pennsylvania, and elsewhere could once again watch their precious offspring fledge the nest, eventually surrendering them to the infinite skies. They still do today.

There is a live-stream eagle cam, active since 2005, located at the U.S. Fish & Wildlife Service's National Conservation Training Center in Shepherdstown,

West Virginia.[9] When I visit the web page one evening in early December and discover no one is home, I am relieved. I used to think that the only people who sit around watching wildlife cams are the same quirky characters who feed dog food to raccoons and celebrate the birthdays of the pandas at the zoo, but I leave the tab open on my desktop. About a month later, at dusk, I check again, and although the nest blows a bit in the wind, it remains empty. This time, I hesitate to admit that I'm a little disappointed.

The next morning, I find two eagles sitting in the bole, the center of the nest, moving sticks around with their beaks. It's not unlike watching beavers find the perfect spot for each branch as they build their dam. At one point the eagles both lift, move, and place the same stick, beaks on opposite ends, like Lady and the Tramp with a strand of spaghetti. It's such an intimate moment, and it's therapeutic to observe nature going about the business of mating without a fuss. (Well, until the webcam watchers observe siblicide, the practice of a larger nest mate killing their eaglet sibling in competition for food.[10])

✳ ✳ ✳

Maybe one day I'll know more about my own reproduction than I do about the effect of DDT on bird eggs, but for now I'll surrender to the present. While I never could have imagined how hard it was to deal with infertility until I experienced it, there is a silver lining. My experiences with "unexplained infertility" invited me to learn more about my animal body than I ever knew before. I learned about the intricacies of a monthly drama playing out below my belly button that was previously a mystery. I learned to tune into my body enough to feel myself ovulating. I explored what foods and exercises support me in different phases of my cycle and how hormones affect my emotional state given the time of month. I thought about other animals' experiences of reproduction and wondered if eagles felt pain when they laid an egg, if they craved a certain fishy flavor during incubation, or if they anticipated the first tiny hole appearing on their tennis-ball-sized egg.

In *Rewilding: Meditations, Practices, and Skills for Awakening in Nature*, Micah Mortali wrote, "Breathe into whatever may be happening right now rather than distracting yourself from it. In many Indigenous cultures, this level of consciousness is associated with birds who soar."[11] Indeed, around the world eagles are associated with kings and consciousness, authority and power, strength and vision.[12] They are sacred to the Navajo[13] and revered as the leader of the birds by the Kanien'kehá:ka people.[14] They are even admired in pop culture as we sing John Denver tunes about eagles around campfires and dance like them to Nelly hits from the early 2000s.

The eagle yoga pose, *garudasana*, is associated not only with an animal but also with a god named Garuda,[15] described as having a golden body, white face, red wings, talons, and a curved beak.[16] He reigns as king of the birds in Hindu mythology and symbolizes integrity because he once carried the nectar of immortality in his beak without drinking a drop of what was not rightfully his.[17] Indonesia's national airline is named after Garuda, and I assure you it feels safer to fly in a plane named after an eagle deity than in one named after a terrestrial creature (sorry, Lion Air)!

As a kid, I had flying dreams that felt so real I was convinced I could simply will myself into the air upon waking and rubbing away my eye boogers. Strangely, I was never disappointed that it didn't work because I was still caught up in the enchantment of the dream. I could close my eyes and continue to sense the wonder of flight as I looked down at the grass and clay of the neighborhood softball fields. But we do not fly in garudasana. In fact, the pose mimics the part of the Ramayana, the seventh-century Hindu epic poem, in which Lord Rama of Ayodhya is attacked, wrapped in snakes during battle, and rescued by Garuda. According to Devdutt Pattanaik, "This is yet another example of why avoiding generic labels like 'eagle pose' is so important. Knowing the story behind the name gives depth to the practice and inspires one to seek further understanding of its origins."[18]

Eagles are not only associated with snakes in Hindu mythology. Understanding animal behavior and ecology, other kinds of stories about the critters we embody, can infuse our practice with meaning. Encounters between eagles and snakes occur in natural predator–prey interactions in which eagles eat snakes and snakes snack on eagle eggs. (Say that 108 times fast!) There is a group of raptors called serpent eagles that live in Asian forests and hunt along habitat edges and adjacent open spaces for snakes, lizards, and small mammals.[19] Meanwhile, African snake eagles catch highly venomous cobras and mambas, tear off their heads, and consume them headfirst, soaring all the while. Individual beyond-human beings are sustained by the foods they consume, and populations are sustained by cycles of reproduction and predation, birth and death. I once observed a Sulawesi serpent eagle and remember nothing of the sighting, although I scribbled the date and general location into my field guide. I surrender to the lost memory, knowing that every eagle I've ever encountered contributes something, however minor, to my idea of them as beyond-human beings today. Even the eagles we forget leave the impressions of their wingbeats on our hearts.

✳ ✳ ✳

Before garudasana we are open and loose. In it, we twist and shrink and pull into ourselves, bound by serpents. Standing on one bent leg, another slithers around it to hook toes around calf in a tenuous bind. Arms intertwine like a self-hug knotted with hesitation. Shoulders strain, hips sink, balance falters. Elbows float imperceptibly toward the clouds. Some people experience that the entwined nature of the pose inspires focus, vision, and purpose,[20] or the feeling of fascia holding their body together and keeping it all connected.[21]

Although garudasana may strengthen and stretch the legs, create opening for tight shoulders, and improve balance,[22] some people wish for it to be over as soon as it begins. Even when we are careful and kind with our bodies during an asana practice, when we are honest with ourselves, sometimes the best part of a pose is the end of it. We release with relief. We "return to openness."[23] We unwind and untangle ourselves because we cannot receive new things all scrunched up like that. Garudasana is less about the form of an eagle (or snake-bound warrior) and more about the release, the changing of energy, the transition from one way of being to another. From imprisoned to liberated. From earth to sky. From hope to surrendering to the discomfort, then back again to hope.

Andrew Schelling wrote about hope from a unique perspective in his essay "Bardo of Lost Mammals" from the book titled *Wild Form, Savage Grammar:*

Poetry, Ecology, Asia, in which I wildly and savagely underlined, drew hearts, and scribbled notes as I read. Thinking of *bardo* as the Buddhist equivalent of the Christian limbo, or a state of spiritual in-betweenness, Schelling suggests the following: 1) Hope is based on the belief that all beings will accompany us on the "Great Journey." The eagles and I, in a sense, have a shared experience of infertility. Although our realities are different in so many ways, none of us is alone. 2) Hope means accepting impermanence. This state in which we find ourselves now will not last forever—it is just one minute, one week, one year, or one lifetime. Even moments of destruction, despair, and suffering can inspire hope because they do not foretell the future. The piece concludes, "With some hard, intelligent work—by eco-activists, biologists, game wardens, Buddhist practitioners, and poets—this might not have to be a hell for some notable species, but a bardo. An in-between state."[24]

While I struggle with hoping for certain things outside of my immediate control, I have an infinite supply of subtle, universal hope for the future of this planet. This kind of hope, according to author Lyanda Lynn Haupt, "involves a willingness to allow that brokenness and beauty sometimes intertwine."[25] It requires our "participation in the renewal of the earth, however that will manifest."[26] It took decades to uncover an explanation for the problem of plummeting eagle populations and reveal the problem of DDT. We used it, then eventually realized its harmful effects and stopped using it. This doesn't mean that we no longer harm animals with dangerous chemicals. It means there was destruction and surrender followed by hope and renewal.

In the context of modern society in the West and the state of our collective relationship with nature, we are currently very snake entangled. That means that change is coming. Freedom is inevitable. Only after we process the tough stuff and open ourselves back up can we conceive of new ways of thinking and being, and most sacred of all, creating new beings. We can surrender for now but hold onto hope that the energy will transition again, away from the snake-bound and terrifying current destruction of the earth to an open and life-nurturing future.

Barbara Ann Kipfer wrote, "We all start life with an eagle and a dove inside us. The eagle is strong and decisive; the dove is peaceful and nurturing. As we grow in maturity, the two birds coalesce into one."[27] I assume that in motherhood, also, the two coalesce into one, like those T-shirts that say "Mama Bear" with the silhouette of a fearsome grizzly beneath dainty, cursive script. My own mountain momma, and all the best mothers I know, are both strong and gentle, fierce and nurturing. I can be two things, too. The eagle in me offers the courage to surrender to the heartbreak and the waiting, to keep arranging the sticks in my nest despite the uncertainty. And the dove inside me dares to hope for an untangled future while remaining mindful in the meantime. Eggshells may have been broken, but my body is not. I unravel my limbs and soften my birdy body.

Practice

BIRD LIKE BUDDHA

1. Observe a single, individual bird. Forget past encounters. Experience the animal in front of you, separate from all previously held knowledge and everything else you long to learn.

2. Abandon the urge to go-go-go, to see more birds. Instead of striking lines through names on a list, yearn to forge a deeper connection with a fellow being.

3. Make your goal to maximize the length of your encounter with this birdy being so you can prioritize the meaning made from this encounter.

4. Try not to name this bird or compare him to another. Let go of your attachment to species names and identifying features. Why does *naming* so often mean "knowing" anyway? Is correctly identifying eight hundred species better than having intimately known a handful?

5. Acknowledge and question your biases suggesting that one bird is "better" than another because she is more "attractive" or less commonly seen. No bird is too common or too drab, or doesn't belong.

6. What does *this* bird look like? Pay attention to the colors, shapes, and textures in front of you.

7. What does *this* bird sound like? Close your eyes and listen.

8. What is *this* bird doing? Catch everything you can about the movements and behaviors of this fellow creature.

9. Imagine yourself as this bird. What would you feel, think, fear, enjoy?

10. Scribble notes, draw sketches, snap photographs, write poems. Consider how you and this bird are sharing space in this world right now. Where is the overlap between human and avian being?

11. Practice nonattachment as the bird floats, flits, dives, or waddles away.

12. Be a perpetually amateur birder.

If birding of any variety is not your jam, become a wildlife camera watcher, if only for a few moments. Check out NCTC's Eagle Cam[28] or explore any number of the zoo and wildlife cams on YouTube. I've enjoyed the Kansas City Zoo Penguin Cam and used it to teach animal behavior methods classes. People also love the Giant Panda Cam at the Smithsonian's National Zoo, and the Monterey Bay Aquarium has a live Jellyfish Cam accompanied by soothing music. Observe individual animals, how they move, and how they transition from one behavior to another. In what ways do they surrender to other individuals or to their surroundings? How does a swimming penguin, a panda munching on bamboo, or an eagle sitting on sticks give you hope?

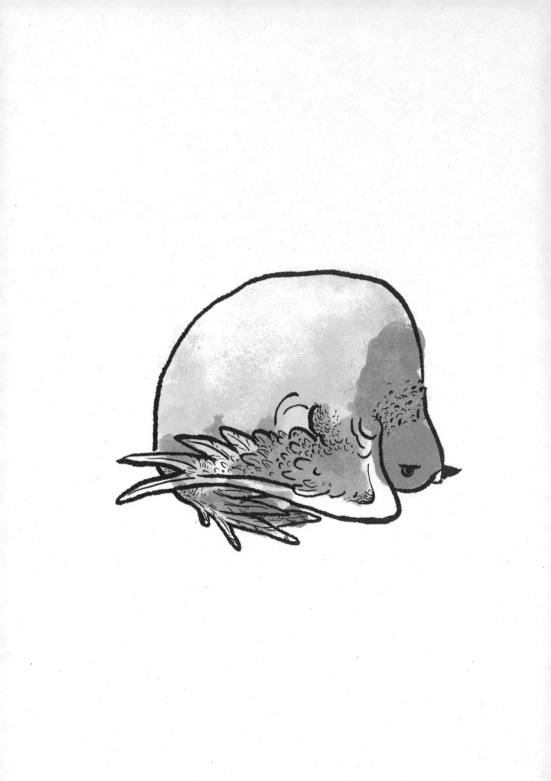

Chapter 3

KAPOTA—PIGEON

Don't move on my yoga mat for three whole minutes? I'll try my best. Squat on a hill in a thorny bush with my neck at a decidedly un-yogic angle watching a fox stalk a rabbit? Twenty minutes, no problem! Although I struggle when my own yoga teacher suggests complete stillness in a restorative pose, I am a statue when I watch wildlife. As Shreve Stockton wrote, "I have a poor concept of time as it is, which disintegrates completely when I'm in the presence of a baby fox."[1] Sometimes I forget to breathe.

The mourning dove perched on my balcony railing is close enough that, through the sliding glass door, I can see her breathe, blink, doze, and swallow. Her tail twitches ever so slightly in time with her breath. A steady breath—not too shallow, not too deep. A balanced, mindful breath. I am close enough to love her as an individual. It's not mourning dove love. It's *this* dove love. Even if she poops on my potted arugula.

She settles deeper into rest, head gently bobbing before appearing to melt down her back as her chest floofs. She faces away from me, then toward me, then away again. I inch closer. She blinks in slow motion. Occasionally, her beak twitches. Her feet are invisible, her flight feathers perfectly scalloped with halos of cream. I want to dissolve the smudged glass door between us.

When I look up from writing in my notebook, she is staring straight at me. *Dictate your soul to me, little dove, and stare as I scribble until your avian heart's content.* She tilts her head.

Someone shouts in the courtyard below and her head emerges a bit from the floof. Even when she faces the opposite direction, I sense her watching me with those prey eyes. When my dog's collar jingles, I jump, startled. I too have a prey mind, I guess. I am becoming prey-er. Prayer flags flutter gently to our left.

I already fear the flapping of her wings so intensely I hear their characteristic whistle in my imagination. How will I feel when she leaves? Where will she go? And why, oh why, would I rather worry about her flying away than enjoy the rise and fall of the feathers right in front of me?

My pen hits the glass, accidentally. She looks at me dead on, and for the first time she is more goofy than cute. I love her even more. My posture slumps as my soul sinks into being with a dove. I have no idea how much time has passed. Ten minutes? Twenty?

Inch by creaking inch I open the sliding glass door and inhale fresh autumn air. I can move more quickly now and make bigger movements without disturbing her, and when I wave away a mosquito she doesn't flinch.

Clumsily, I back into a potted aloe plant that scratches my arm as dirt spills onto the hardwood floor. (I won't sweep it up for days.) I slide onto my belly and pop my head out the door. My hand cradles my chin the way her wings fold against her body.

I smile. She blinks. I blink.

Then she begins the mourning dove shuffle. It goes like this: tail preen, wing stretch, shuffle right, head bob, repeat. Throw in a throat flutter and set to a sassy tune.

My heart beats faster.

She is completely still, almost a silhouette in the falling dusk.

I sigh.

She shuffles left, stretches her wings one at a time, nibbles her foot, bobs her head, and flies away. I rush outside to feel the metal banister where her warm bird feet perched, but it is already cold.

❊ ❊ ❊

I have encountered doves and pigeons, alive and quite dead, around the world. I observed eared doves strutting down the streets of Quito, peaceful doves atop headstones in a Muslim cemetery in Borneo, spotted doves in Bali, and rock doves on statues throughout Europe and across the U.S. Once in Hyderabad, India, I got out of the car with my mother-in-law to shop for jewelry and realized with a jolt that she was about to step on a pigeon carcass lying in the gutter. It was too late for me to warn her, she didn't notice,

and I decided not to tell her. Back in the car after a failed search for the perfect pair of party earrings, I whispered about the dead bird to my husband,
Vishu. He chuckled and told his mom, who immediately became upset and
understandably grossed out. I swatted at Vishu for bringing it up, but he
was laughing harder now. From the driver's seat, my father-in-law sang a
cheerful Bollywood tune as he navigated the city's eternal traffic.

"It's a song about a pigeon," Vishu explained.

In the rearview mirror, my father-in-law's eyes were smiling.

There are many members of the Columbidae family, of which pigeons and
mourning doves are a part, whom I still yearn to encounter in the wild. I want
to behold the bright green wings of emerald doves, of course, but also their
little orange beaks that resemble the carrot noses of only the jolliest of snow-
people. In Papua New Guinea, Victoria crowned pigeons wear nature's most
flamboyant headpieces and dance across the forest floor. Meanwhile in Asia
and the Pacific islands, fruit doves masquerade as regal parrots.

While we may not think twice about seeing a mourning dove or feral
pigeon, these birds live out fascinating lives in our cities and backyards,
some for lifespans of over thirty years. They are mostly ground feeders,
although compared with doves, pigeons tend to forage more in trees and
flock in larger groups. They walk upon the earth with a certain distinction,
bobbing their heads and rhythmically strutting like marionette puppets.
The Sibley Guide to Birds suggests that members of the Columbidae family
"fly like falcons" and "walk like turkeys."[2] A winning combo! They are also
cognitively impressive, capable of learning and recalling patterns, sharing
attention, using tools, remembering images, and discriminating between
individuals. In one famous study, scientists trained pigeons to differentiate
between Picasso and Monet paintings.[3]

Have you ever looked—really looked—at a mourning dove? My field
guide describes the species as small-headed, slender, and sandy or fawn-
colored, with bluish shading, long wings, and a long tail that inspired the
Latin species name, *macroura*.[4] One difference between males and females
is a princely, pinkish hue to the male's breast—which was never more obvious
than the day, early in the coronavirus lockdown, when Vishu and I ogled
a pair mating in the courtyard below. Another admirable trait, noted in

proverb and poetry throughout the ages, is the devotion that mourning doves display toward their mates.

Not everyone writes with such fondness for the mourning dove, though. Neltje Blanchan, author of a book about birds from 1904, described doves as incessant and melancholy with a dirge-like song and poor parental skills. Commenting on maternal behavior, she wrote with needless aggression: "She is a flabby, spineless bundle of flesh and pretty feathers, gentle and refined in manners, but slack and incompetent in all she does. . . . We are almost inclined to blame the inconsiderate mother for allowing her offspring to enter the world unclothed—obviously not her fault, though she is capable of just such negligence."[5] Yikes.

In fact, doting dove mothers go so far as to partially digest their babies' food and regurgitate it directly into their waiting beaks. (It's called pigeon milk. *Yum.*) The nestlings are called squabs, an appropriately goofy moniker for the little dinosaurs-in-training who sit in sparse nests upon haphazardly placed sticks. Yes, dove nests may be considered minimalist in style, but their reproductive success has hardly suffered from it. Although mourning doves are some of the most common birds in North America, birders from other parts of the world delight in their sightings the way I might cherish a glimpse of the jewel-toned Nicobar pigeon.

We've all heard the mourning dove's song, but it surprised me how often in my work guiding nature hikes that adults and children alike would hear it in the middle of the day and ask, "Is that an owl?" Males seeking a mate emit soft "perch-coos" from a prominent spot on a branch. In my memory, my brother brings his fingernail-nibbled hand to his mouth and imitates the five notes to near perfection. *Coo-OO! Oo-oo-oo....*

Pigeons are the larger and more disdained members of family Columbidae, if you can believe it given Blanchan's harsh critique of the mourning dove. Introduced to North America in the 1600s, these chunky, red-eyed, white-rumped city birds now thrive in urban areas and utter their guttural coos among honking horns and smog. Although there is no clear taxonomic distinction between doves and pigeons, many humans favor one over the other. A rock dove and a feral pigeon both poop on the same street corner (indeed, they are the same bird), yet the two names evoke quite different creatures.

There are many proposed reasons for popular human hatred of the common pigeon, also known as rats or cockroaches with wings and flying ashtrays. In the 1950s, there was concern that pigeons spread disease, but these accusations are unfounded.[6] Others claim they damage property and displace native birds; yet, while a single bird can excrete approximately twenty-five pounds of poop per year, sociologist Colin Jerolmack suggests that people hate pigeons not because of anything the birds do but because they represent nature thriving in a place some modern minds are unwilling to allow. He argues that "pigeons have come to represent the antithesis of the ideal metropolis, which is orderly and sanitized, with nature subdued and compartmentalized."[7] Nature, to many, still belongs "out there" where the pavement turns to dirt, honking horns become birdsong, and stoplights are starlight. We are uncomfortable sharing such intimacy—our road rage and dropped French fries—with feral pigeons. A dove, on the other hand, olive branch betwixt beak, symbolizes love, peace, hope, and the Holy Spirit. The pooping pigeon perched on a park bench cannot compete with our ideas of divine doves.

In fact, because they are strong fliers with impressive homing behaviors, pigeons have been used to help humans communicate for millennia. Long before the postal service, telephones, and the internet, carrier pigeons were trained to fly hundreds of miles, deliver messages, and return to their home roost. They can see, smell, hear, and navigate the world better than we can. Pigeons have monocular vision with a 340-degree field of view compared to our measly 120 degrees. They can see ultraviolet light and hear infrasound frequencies beyond our sensing ability. Pigeons not only excelled in art class but also served as war heroes. Thanks to these physical and behavioral adaptations, famous birds named Cher Ami, President Wilson, G.I. Joe, and Commando delivered messages amidst raging battles and saved the lives of soldiers and civilians alike in World Wars I and II.

✳ ✳ ✳

There are as many versions of *kapotasana* as there are pigeons in the world (i.e., a lot). *Kapota* means "dove" or "pigeon" because in the pose, "the chest is pushed forward like that of a pouter pigeon" according to B.K.S. Iyengar.[8]

In Hindu mythology, Shiva, the god of destruction, took goddess Parvati to a remote Himalayan cave to share the secret of immortality. To ensure their privacy before uttering such sacred words, Shiva burned everything around the cave so no other creature could disturb them. Neither of them realized that two pigeon eggs remained under the deerskin upon which they sat. (Indeed, the wild counterparts of feral pigeons used to live and nest in caves and cliffs.) As Shiva spoke, the eggs hatched, and the birds overheard the mantra of immortality. Growing up in Florida, I drank from the Fountain of Youth, but perhaps I should forget Ponce de Leon and ask the pigeons how to stay forever young!

During yoga, we puff out our chests hundreds of times without understanding or embodying this humble bird. In a recent class during which I taught restorative variations of kapotasana, I led students through a quick visualization before we began. In it, they imagined that they were walking through a forest and happened upon a large, beautiful tree with a hollow trunk. When they walked inside there was a soft, glowing light, comfy moss to sit on, and two pigeons.

"Just sit together, you and the pigeons," I instructed, "I want you to encounter the birds whose bodies you are about to mimic. To call their shape and essence to mind. Too often, we think nothing of the animals whose poses we practice."

Kapotasana can be a beneficial pose to counteract the position we find ourselves stuck in for hours on end in daily life—hunched over and on our bums. In office chairs, the seats of cars, and cushions of couches, our bodies fold at the hips as our backs hunch and chests collapse. In the pigeon shape, our hips and hearts open and our backs bend to counter perpetual poor posture. The spine, thighs, buttocks, ankles, and chest may feel stretched and strengthened. Circulation and flexibility, especially in the hips and legs, may improve.[9]

On my own yoga mat, I marvel at the pigeon form as I scrutinize the angle at which my front knee bends while my other leg—I mean my tail—extends behind me, stick straight. Indeed, it helps me balance as it does the feathered and flighted. I fold over my front leg and bow, grounded, no itch to fly. Most days, looking earthward is enough. Sometimes I bend my back knee and wonder about the mechanics of it all. Birds' tails can bend this way, too. If I listen carefully when Monkey, my adopted budgie, preens, I can hear the little barbules of each feather zipping back into place as she pulls the entire length of her lapis blue tail through the hook of her beak. Only rarely, I am *rajakapota*, king pigeon. Bending my back knee and hooking flexed foot into elbow crook, my hands bound, I gaze skyward and imagine the soft whistle of wings.

Being pigeon is easy; becoming pigeon is the challenge. Like my mourning dove neighbor, I, too, wiggle a bit and settle in before taking flight. Left to right. Toes curled, then uncurled, I fidget and experiment with wing and limb. Pigeons are anisodactyl like most perching birds, with one toe in the back and three in the front. I press my fingertips into the floor at the ends of tented hands, three in front, thumb in back, pinky askew. I open my chest and my heart, and gaze toward the waiting sky. The kapotasana shuffle goes like this: roll the shoulders, rock gently side to side, lift and settle back foot, repeat. Throw in a look over each wing before folding forward over the front leg. Set to a languorous tune. Aldo Leopold once wrote that pigeons written about in books "live forever by not living at all."[10] Free the pigeons from this book. Give them life. Move your body. Floof your chest. Be and breathe with pigeons both real and imagined.

I love pigeon pose because it's perfect for practicing nonattachment. One of my favorite quotes, by Eckhart Tolle in *The Power of Now,* is "Forgive yourself for not being at peace."[11] I would like to add: Forgive yourself for not being pigeon. We cannot expect to invoke the birds each and every time we guide our bodies into kapotasana. I don't. We also cannot appreciate every passing pigeon with devoted, mindful attention. That's okay. The tragic fate of the extinct passenger pigeon behind us, resilient rock doves are here to stay. They are not endangered. They are everywhere. Hunters shoot them, birders list them, and the hungry eat them. My great-grandfather raised pigeons above his garage after immigrating from Slovakia to New Jersey, and my dad remembers taking live birds home to butcher, after which they flew around the basement without heads. Opportunities abound to connect with pigeons (alive, and yes, sometimes dead). As Rosemary Mosco says, "It's a hard world. Sometimes you just need to look at a soft bird."[12] Doves and pigeons are a part of our backyards, cities, and family folklore, for better or worse, now and into an optimistically, coo-filled future.

On yoga mats, in caves, atop skyscrapers . . . we are not alone.

May bird feet warm your banister.

Practice

KAPOTA MUDRA

There is no more perfect *mudra* ("symbolic hand gesture") for cultivating compassion than the feeling of holding a dove between the palms of your hands. Kapota mudra helps us cultivate *ahimsa* ("non-harming"), which radiates from our hearts out to other beings.[13] Doves symbolize peace, which is impossible without ahimsa.

Think of this gesture like an inflated version of Anjali mudra, typical yoga "prayer hands" in which the palms are brought together in front of the chest, fingertips facing up. Sit in a chair, cross-legged on a cushion, or on a folded blanket on the ground. Begin with your hands at your heart, palms together. Keep the tips and sides of your fingers, and inner edges of your thumbs, together as you bend your knuckles and "inflate" your palms while bringing the tips of the thumbs and index fingers toward each other. The shape of your hands should resemble a dove's body. When practicing any mudra, achieving the gist of the shape with comfort is more beneficial than striving toward an "accurate" gesture filled with tension. Breathe naturally, in and out through the nose, as you hold the mudra at your heart. Remember that the divine is as present in the hearts of doves as it is now between and behind your two cupped hands.

Imagine your breath flowing through your own heart and into the hollows of your hands in a sacred exchange of human and bird. Contemplate the small ways you can reduce harm to yourself and others, visualizing the effects of those simple compassionate actions rippling outward in expansive ways, spreading peace. Before your arms tire, relax your hands, palms facing up, onto your legs. Open your eyes.

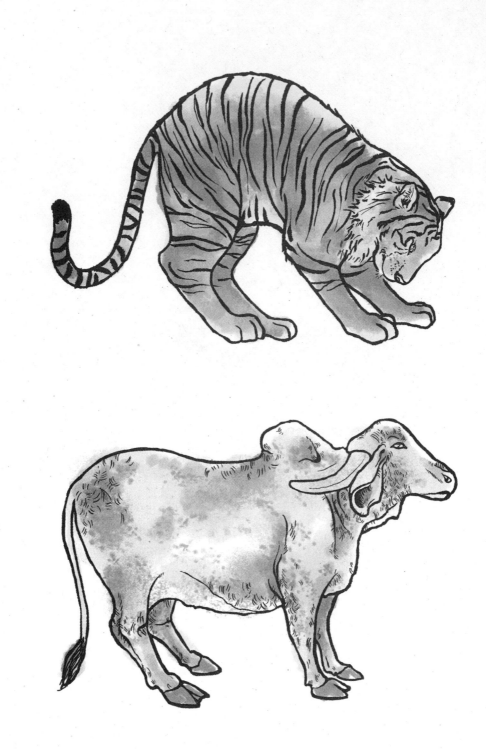

Chapter 4
BIDALA/GO—CAT/COW

Inhale prey....

"Mau lihat?" ("Do you want to watch?")

My friends repeated this question in Indonesian until finally, anxious, I walked from the front porch over to the corral.

The human and beyond-human beings around me seemed stressed and excited, stimulated by an abundance of activity and new smells in the air. In the Islamic tradition, the Qur'an permits animal sacrifice on Eid al-Adha to commemorate Ibrahim's devotion to Allah and his willingness to sacrifice his son, Ismail. In Sulawesi, an island in the Indonesian archipelago, the holiday involves *potong sapi,* which literally translates as "cow cutting." Part of me wanted to observe this ritual that I knew was so important to my Muslim friends, but in the end, I averted my eyes.

Months later at the local university, as I sipped sweet coffee and waited for GIS data to transfer to my flash drive, a professor showed me videos of *potong kerbau* ("buffalo sacrifice") from his recent trip home to Tana Toraja, another part of the island, to celebrate the holiday. I stared at the corner of his laptop screen staving off a panic attack. *Tidak mau lihat.* Again, I didn't want to watch. I saw out of the corner of my eye that the video was paused as a long blade met the neck of the buffalo. The animal was understandably panicked after having already seen four of his kind meet the same fate.

A couple of people gathered in the small office and stood around my chair, watching.

"He could probably smell their blood," someone said.

As the video resumed, the buffalo thrashed around for a few minutes, bleeding from the throat.

Soon after this stressful, peripheral viewing of the Torajan buffalo sacrifice, back at my field site I watched the 2011 film *Samsara* with my primatology colleagues. It included footage from factory farms in North America that "produced" chickens, cows, and pigs. It was suddenly so obvious: If I were a *sapi*, I would much prefer a life wandering the Sulawesi countryside, grazing in the sunshine, mating by the night light of camera traps, and experiencing a few moments of suffering at death, compared to enduring a lifetime of cruelty by Americans who treat certain animals like nonliving commodities.

Potong sapi is only one example of animal sacrifice from a particular region. Within Islam, a lot of variation exists in the role animals play in religious practices. I recently read about the Van Gujjars, a community of Muslim, historically migratory buffalo herders in the Himalayas, who are traditionally averse to consuming the animals they raise.[1] In *Animal Intimacies*, Radhika Govindrajan wrote about goat sacrifice in India:

> The death of an animal with whom people feel embodied kinship creates a sense of loss and grief that is essential to making sacrifice truly a sacrifice.... At the heart of all such gestures was an acknowledgment that one's life was intertwined with that of another and that this connection implied some responsibility on the part of those who were alive to those who were or would soon be dead, especially because that death was intended to benefit the living.[2]

We must remember that, when a sacrifice is truly a sacrifice, loss, sometimes heartbreak, is experienced. When we remove ourselves from the act of the sacrifice, ritual or not, we lose out on the connection and responsibility that accompanies using and consuming the bodies and products of other beings for the sake of religion, nutrition, or any other reason. In the end, it is not the meat and blood that matters to Allah or any other deity—it is the intention within the heart of the one who sacrifices.

And what of the nonhuman animal's experience? Is there any part of the sacrifice that is not characterized by fear and suffering for the animal?

Considering that relationships between people and other animals are often reciprocal, we should leave room for some sort of meaning. I'm not suggesting that animals consent to their own sacrifice, but if it means so much to the humans with whom their lives were entangled, there may be something else going on. I consider the possibility that my own fear of witnessing the sacrifice could have somehow caused suffering for the sapi. Maybe if I felt gratitude or faith or compassion instead of anxiety and ignorance, I could have provided some comfort to the animals involved. We may never know, but we can use questions like these to consider additional ways of relating to other beings.

Sacrifice and consumption are also entangled. As Shreve Stockton noted, "Eating is intimacy . . . perhaps, by consuming a cow or a chicken or a celery stalk, all of which must die to feed us, we are meant to be reminded, daily, at the cellular level, of the interconnectedness of everything. That, in fact, nothing is separate; everything is linked. That we are a part of it, that we are made of it."[3] Maybe this was Allah's plan all along. Throughout my twenties I went from being an ominovore to being a pescatarian to eating meat only if I didn't personally create the demand for it.

Then one day about four years ago, scrolling on my phone while waiting for my bubble tea order, I came across an article about a farm sanctuary in New York that offers rescue turkeys their own Thanksgiving feast. There were pictures of the turkeys eating veggies, fruits, and pumpkin pie at a table set with fancy dishes and dressed with a tablecloth. There was something about that simple idea of a Thanksgiving meal turned on its head. As I stood in line with BTS blaring, I finally admitted that while enjoying the occasional turkey sandwich might satisfy me for approximately two minutes, eating according to my principles and living my compassion for other beings might ultimately make me a happier, more authentic version of myself. Now, I am a vegetarian who occasionally cheats.

In Indonesia, following the events of potong sapi, families and communities gather together in new outfits to enjoy elaborate feasts. Meat and other foods are generously shared with those who are unable to afford the sacrifice themselves. Once, it was shared with a non-Muslim researcher from the U.S. who wanted to avoid the heartbreak of the loss of a life and

still consume the spicy, coconutty, delicious result. As I chewed on my beef
rendang that night six years ago, I regretted not having the courage to watch.

✳ ✳ ✳

. . . exhale predator.

"This is where I have seen many leopards," said our guide, Sanju, as we
walked down the hillside to our campsite. My husband and I were visiting
Great Himalayan National Park, and it was the final night of our six-day
honeymoon trek. The forest canopy above us was so dense it felt like the
sun had already set.

Sanju pointed out a place on the side of the trail where the dirt and vegetation had been recently disturbed. It reminded me of the aftermath of wild
pigs foraging in the sandy Florida soil.

"A leopard chased a goral here three hours ago," he said, referring to the
common goat-antelope critters that roam alone or in small herds in lower
elevations of the park.

"Have leopards ever attacked a person here?" I asked, recalling many
scholarly articles about human–carnivore conflict in the subcontinent.

"Not that I know of," Sanju responded.

One fictionalized account of the Ramayana describes the first instance
of what we now call human–wildlife conflict. It took place in India when a
tigress attacked a child out of revenge because someone from that village
hunted one of her cubs.[4] There is still conflict today between humans and
large cats throughout the world. In the Sundarbans in Bangladesh, people
fear for their lives in the mangroves where they work, sometimes wearing
masks with eyes on the backs of their heads to deceive tigers. At one tiger
reserve in Central India, 132 people were attacked by tigers and leopards
over the span of seven years. More than half of those attacks were deadly,
and the most dangerous context in which the attacks occurred was when
people were collecting forest resources far from the village.[5]

Generally, leopards are a more common problem than tigers in India
because there are more of them, and because they are more adaptable to
human-inhabited spaces. They live at the edges of different habitats, between
forests and villages, around towns, and even near cities. A single leopard

reportedly killed 125 people over the span of a decade in Rudraprayag, and from 2000 to 2016 there were 159 reported leopard attacks in the Pauri Garhwal district of Uttarakhand, many of them on children.[6] Wildlife biologists suspect that many attacks occur here because the abandoned terraced hills provide ample cover for leopards to hide and hunt. Wandering livestock and, tragically, sometimes children, are easy prey. Despite the fear of coexisting with large cats, the people in these places tend to admire and worship the beyond-human beings who may threaten their lives. In the Indian Sundarbans the tiger god Dakshin Ray is praised and thanked for the natural riches that the mangrove forests provide to local people.[7]

While the behavior of "man-eating" cats can be explained by a wide variety of circumstances ranging from religion to retaliation, there are also reasons that relate to the life history and natural habitat of the animals. In the same way that observing and thinking about wildlife enables us to connect with nature through our asana practice, understanding the ecological explanations behind large cat behavior can contribute considerable insight to addressing human conflicts. Population size and density, age, health, preferred habitat, availability of wild prey, individual cat behavior, human behavior, time of year, and proximity to protected areas and human settlements may all at some point influence whether or not a leopard or tiger attacks a person.[8] For example, sometimes large cats attack people not to eat them, but to defend themselves if they have been cornered or if they perceive that their young are threatened. A large cat who is old or sick and no longer a successful hunter might also seek easier prey to survive.

Wild cats are usually more of a threat to livestock than to people. In central India leopards and tigers may threaten herds of buffalo and cattle, and in Nepal snow leopards kill the occasional yak. In places where conflict mitigation has been most successful, social scientists, ecologists, and community leaders work together to address these problematic examples of human–wildlife interaction.[9] Sometimes, compensation programs provide financial support to ranchers who experience livestock loss. In other areas, nonlethal methods such as guardian dogs, fences, and blowing flags are used to protect livestock and the cats who may be tempted to feast upon them.[10]

Back in the Himalayan forest, the three of us stopped short in the middle of the trail.

"That's the smell of a leopard," Sanju said.

The scent resembled musky popcorn and hung heavy in the air, strong and distinct. When we finally reached camp as daylight faded, Sanju pointed to a large boulder not far from our tent.

"That's where a leopard once scared some tourists from Mumbai," he laughed.

Although we smelled leopard twice more that afternoon, we never saw one.

✳ ✳ ✳

My encounters with felines have been only fleeting. If birders "count" birds they only hear singing, then I suppose I have encountered a leopard by smelling it. I am torn; the experience of the cat's scent was both enough and not nearly enough. I've never seen a wild cat of any kind, although bobcats and mountain lions have surely seen me. My dad is allergic to cats, so I never had the experience of childhood feline companionship. I suspect I have practiced the cat yoga pose more times than I have met real live cats, wild or domestic.

"Arch your back like a Halloween cat," says my yoga teacher as we kneel on hands and knees, tuck chins to chests, and drop tailbones toward the earth.

A Halloween cat is not exactly what I have in mind. What makes a cat a cat, anyway? They are all carnivorous, clawed (hopefully), and curious. Some are social and others are solitary. Some cats roar and others say, "O Most Compassionate One" with every purr, according to Turkish Sufi teacher Bediuzzaman Said Nursi, who understood the language of animals.[11] Cat pose, called *bidalasana,* can be great for spine mobility and works muscles in the back and the abdomen. Typically, it is practiced with the exhale because the movement decreases lung volume.[12]

After cat pose inevitably comes cow pose, the weight of a full udder guiding our bellies toward the earth. This pair of animals is forever linked by yoga. I've never practiced cat without cow or vice versa. To do one without the other is like . . . well, inhaling without exhaling. The two poses are like a strange yogic version of those stories of animal friendships between a cheetah and a dog or a lioness and a baby antelope. In our bodies, as well as in a very real ecological sense, there is no cat without cow, no leopard without goral. We flex and arch our backs, moving our spines in fluid animal undulations, all while kneeling on four limbs, experiencing what it's like to be a quadruped, a four-limbed creature. Denise Kaufman wrote, "Perhaps as humans we need to reclaim our four-leggedness."[13]

The flow from cat to cow could also be interpreted as the comparison between wild and domestic. For me, the word *domesticated* conjures images of livestock or pets. The two most common pets are dogs and cats according to a 2018 survey conducted by the American Veterinary Medical Association. In the online version of the *Merriam-Webster Dictionary*, the process of animal domestication occurs over time through selective breeding, resulting in proximity to and benefits for humans.

Scientific research backs up my hunch based on anecdotes from bemused cat caregivers that their pets are not really that domesticated. If they are, it occurred within the last two centuries, although they have lived near and among humans for much longer. "It is probably more accurate to view *Felis catus* as a subspecies that has drifted unpredictably in and out of various states of domestication, semi-domestication and feralness depending on the particular ecological and cultural conditions prevailing at different times and locations," wrote James A. Serpell.[14] Pet cats, even the ones who spend their entire lives within the walls of someone's home, regularly remind their human companions that they are wild, independent thinkers. They act domesticated selectively and on their own terms.

While I am wary of dichotomies like human–animal and wild–domestic, humor me for a moment. Imagine a spectrum with *wild* on one end and *domesticated* on the other. Where would you fall? Regardless of your answer, a transition from the wild, a tending toward the domestic, is a relatable concept as our lives become increasingly sedentary, predictable, and indoors. A wild asana practice moves the needle back in the other direction. Even house cats nudge us toward remembering our wild with a purr and then a hiss, a swat of the paw at a moth in the night, or a gentle kneading to awaken us the next morning. Cows also live intriguing individual lives if we let them be a bit wild. For example, at Rosamund Young's Kite's Nest Farm in England, where the cows all have space to roam, her family observed that they are happier, healthier, and more intelligent because of it.[15] Our yoga practice is one of the simple things we can do to claim more wildness in our own bodies, minds, and lives.

✳ ✳ ✳

When we practice asana, we partner with animals to keep our spines flexible and to keep us agile and wild. Farmers partner with cats called mousers for pest control that prevents crop loss and contamination. Ranchers partner with cattle to protect and improve soil quality and promote native plant growth. Eccentric, crafty folks even have creative partnerships with their pet cats as they knit or felt with the hair their pets shed. In a sense, tigers and people partner to protect each other's space and safety when the fear of one (the cats) keeps the other (the people) from "disturbing" the forests in which they live.

While I may not have a cat in my home, I have traveled to the Malaysian "City of Cats," named Kuching (the Bahasa Malay word for "cat"), where people partner with felines. While tourists snap selfies next to way-larger-than-life-sized cat statues and visit the world's first cat museum, locals of Chinese, Malay, Indian, and tribal origin feed strays and honor the convergence of cultures that manifests in the form of feline appreciation.[16] When we partner with other animals we are better together, practically and spiritually.

There is much to learn from the ways deities partner with animals like cats and cows. In the Hindu tradition, many of the gods and goddesses partner with beyond-human beings. Revered animals assisted the divine and became known as *vahanas*, "vehicles," to the gods. For example, Saraswati, the goddess of knowledge, sits atop a swan. Ganesha, the elephant-headed god who removes obstacles, rides a mouse, and Shiva perches astride a bull named Nandi. The animals not only closely resemble species still roaming the earth; they were historically sacred, totemic figures who were incorporated into what is now recognized as the Hindu pantheon.[17]

The goddess known popularly as Durga is Mother of the Universe and the embodiment of the Divine Feminine. Ruler of all creatures and provider for beings in need. Great warrior and slayer of the buffalo demon Mahishasura. And she does it all with a tiger vahana. Durga's vehicle is feline. Some say there are two sides to the Goddess, "the malevolent as well as the benevolent one. Nature can be cruel and kind."[18] I believe there are more than two sides to the Goddess. Perhaps her cat's fabled nine lives represent her different forms: creator, preserver, destroyer, nurturer, warrior, healer, protector, liberator, and partner. The word *feline* itself feels like a sacred blending, a partnership between the *feminine* and the *divine.* Cats are indeed associated with the mother goddess, as they embody maternal instincts to both fiercely protect and tenderly nurture their young.[19] If the divine feminine represents nature in contrast to the masculine representation of the mind, by having a cat as her vehicle, Durga "defies domestication"[20] as many "cat people" observe their own pets doing.

There is some confusion as to what kind of cat, exactly, is Durga's animal partner. Neither a house cat with a neon fishbone collar, to be sure, nor a feral street cat with nicked ears and darting eyes. A quick survey of the top twenty web search results for *Durga* depicts the goddess seated atop a tiger in six pictures and a lion in fourteen.

"So, which is it?" I ask my Hindu mother-in-law.

"Tiger," she says, after which we discuss where each of the big cats live and the current status of their populations in India.

Many people are surprised to learn there are lions in Asia in addition to Africa. The endangered Asiatic lion's range is limited to the state of Gujarat, and there are fewer than a thousand individuals left.[21] Tigers have fared a bit better. There are an estimated three thousand Bengal tigers in India, and not too many more globally,[22] but populations have increased in recent years.[23] Zoologist K. Ullas Karanth suggests that the success of tiger conservation in the country is due, in part, to the role of the tiger in India's religion, mythology, and folklore in addition to modern marketing and pride in the country's official national animal.[24]

"Even if all the animals go extinct, Durga will ride a truck or something," my mother-in-law concludes.

She delivers the statement in a joking tone, but it's a poignant commentary on wildlife conservation and religion, referring to both the impermanence of nature and the resilience of Hindu tradition. In one sense, when tigers eat the animals they are "supposed" to eat (deer instead of people, pets, or livestock, as that concept is defined by humans), they control prey populations, creating somewhat of an ecological "balance" much like the equilibrium that was restored on earth after Durga's defeat of the deceitful buffalo demon. It is no coincidence that Durga and her tiger defeat a bovine buffalo. After all, buffaloes are relatives of cattle and common prey of large, wild cats. Mythology mirrors nature.

On the other hand, a tiger need not be defined only by its temporary, earthly identity as predator. According to stories from Hindu holy places such as Rishi Agastya's hermitage (the ashram of a revered sage) and Mount Kailash (a sacred Tibetan peak), tigers and goats play together in a realm where there is no predator, no prey, and no hunger.[25] I try to imagine a world in which the cow does not fear the big cat, in which the goral does not flee the leopard while traversing steep Himalayan trails littered with candy wrappers, but I struggle to understand the implications of such a reordering. I was taught the inevitability of predator–prey relationships from a young age: from the horror film music that plays (to my utter rage) during every nature documentary chase scene to the red-shouldered hawk who ate the tufted titmouse fledgling in my backyard as I watched from the window.

It is a challenge to consider that such examples of predator–prey friendship might not be as rare as we think. One real-life cat–cow example sparked widespread curiosity in the Vadodara district of Gujarat, India, in the fall of 2002. A farmer lived near a protected area with a population of approximately three hundred leopards. One night, he heard something outside his home and was shocked to discover a female leopard head-butting his cow, who willingly reciprocated, seeming to engage in play. He watched their interactions from a window, in disbelief, as the cat visited the cow multiple times each night and for many nights over the course of a few months.

The leopard was cautious during her nocturnal approaches, wary of people with cameras and flashlights who visited to see for themselves the evidence of this rare friendship. The cow seemed to expect the cat before she arrived. Sometimes they lay down together with their bodies touching; other times the cow licked the leopard's head and neck, a bonding behavior observed in cattle.[26] Occasionally the cat made gurgling noises toward the cow, which were interpreted by human witnesses as submissive vocalizations. The leopard did not act aggressively toward the cow and the cow did not seem to fear the leopard, both reactions we would expect based on our limited understanding of these animals and their assigned roles as either predator or prey.

How and why did this friendship endure? The anonymous author who detailed the phenomenon in a blog post was at a loss for an answer but wrote, "People more knowledgeable than forest officers and field biologists insist that the two animals had shared a close relationship in their previous births. Some priests hinted at a supernatural relationship."[27] I am delighted to consider such alternative explanations, but to science's credit, we do know that cows establish and maintain friendships that are critically important to individual health and well-being. Researchers found that cows who spend time grazing and resting with their preferred companions have lower heart rates and exhibit fewer anxious behaviors such as pacing and head tossing.[28] We don't know the beginning of this story, but the cow knew the leopard as an individual and changed her behavior accordingly. They trusted each other and enjoyed each other's company.

If domesticated cows can tell each other apart and prefer the company of some individuals to others, of course they can distinguish between another prey species and one that could hunt and hurt them. In fact, livestock response to approaching carnivores is a topic of interest among those hoping to mitigate human–wildlife conflict. One research team found that while wild ungulates exhibit more vigilance than cattle domesticated more than ten thousand years ago,[29] cows do scan their surroundings while foraging to watch for predators.[30] By focusing more studies on "the hunted" instead of "the hunter" and learning more about the specific contexts in which increased vigilance is displayed, we can better understand cattle behaviors that might protect them from future attacks. These results may eventually inform more effective prevention of carnivore predation on livestock.

In Durga's story, the bovine villain Mahishasura is the hunted *and* the hunter. He is much more than his buffalo form. He represents the human concept of dominion over nature,[31] an idea undoubtedly linked to domestication. Interestingly, to some people who share space with tigers in Malaysia, adherence to the belief of human dominance over nature is what partially protects them. According to some Muslims in this region, the reason a tiger attacks someone only from behind is because the verse from the Qur'an stating that humans are superior to nature is visible to the tiger on everyone's foreheads.[32] To others, an initial glance at common depictions of certain deities and their "mounts" may suggest dominance over instead of partnership with animals, as the gods appear to ride or control their "vehicles" in an arrangement similar to our own relationships with domesticated horses, for example.

I choose to understand Durga's relationship with her cat as something more nuanced than a goddess riding an animal to dominate and use it. Just as there is no cat pose without cow pose, there is no Durga without her tiger. I partnered with the Goddess one day, unintentionally at first, in the midst of a particularly challenging emotional time. I was listening to a Durga chant—not singing along or meditating or summoning anything. I was lying there enduring the helplessness I felt and suddenly, Durga was beside me. She laid her weapons down on the carpet and sat in peaceful meditation on the floor to my right. I never opened my eyes, but I knew she was with me. I knew the tigress was there too and that her striped body lay in the corner of my little home office in front of an Ikea bookcase. Her watchful eyes shone with both ferocity and care. All would be well. Tears of comfort, relief, and multispecies (and beyond-species!) divine feminine companionship soaked my eye pillow. When the chant ended, I eased out of the pose and rushed downstairs to kneel in front of Durga's image at the altar where, the day before, I had placed fresh marigolds that grew in a pot on our front steps. I touched my forehead to the floor beneath the idol, beneath two resin-sculpted goddess feet and four paws etched with tiny lines to mimic the texture of tiger fur.

If this didn't happen to me, I wouldn't believe it. Things like this don't happen to me. Admittedly, the tiger's presence in my home office made a lot more sense to me than a visit from any deity—as I have worshipped animals, in my own way, for far longer than any god or goddess. This visit from Durga and her cat was a reminder, not only that we are never alone but also that the appeal of the Hindu deities especially is that they have experienced the trials of life as we have. From countless mythological examples we know that they have felt sorrow and jealousy and fiery rage. They have needed animals to travel and to win battles both literal and metaphorical. They need animals to save themselves and to save the world.

Studying the relationships between people, cats, cows, and deities in South Asia, the birthplace of yoga, can inspire us and allow us to see more clearly the divinity within us as we consider how gods and goddesses partner with the beings we mimic on our mats. These are often familiar creatures with whom we share physical characteristics, behaviors, ancestors, and the planet. Perhaps you have one in your home now, splayed out and snoozing in a slice of sun coming through the window. Maybe you recently drove past a herd of them, seeking solace in the shade of a pasture's only oak tree. If not, you can still know the power of partnership with the divine. If you can't share your life with a cat or a cow, be a cat and a cow. Get down on your hands and knees. Meow and moo.

"Arch your back like Durga's tigress," I tell my students. "Claw into your mat with tender ferocity."

"Now, drop your belly like a Sulawesi sapi. Roam the beautiful countryside. Replace your hands with hooves."

Inhale prey.

Exhale predator.

Practice

CAT/COW BREATH EXCHANGE

Come down onto your hands and knees and place a folded blanket under your knees for cushioning. If you prefer, you can do this same exercise seated on the edge of a chair, away from the chair back to give your spine and torso plenty of space to move and explore. From either position, make sure your spine is long and neutral, and spend a minute focused on your breath. You don't have to change your natural breathing in any way. If you start to think about something else, notice it, and return your attention to your breath.

Let your body start to move with your breath. Better yet, let your breath move your body in intuitive ways. How does your body respond when you inhale versus when you exhale? How does the spine move as the air flows in and out of your body? If it feels comfortable, let the movements become more exaggerated as you warm up. With each inhale, open your heart (physically and metaphorically) and consider that a cow has breathed the very same breath as you—those same molecules of air—yesterday or last century. "This breath, right now, so ancient, yet so fresh," wrote Micah Mortali.[33] With each exhale, arch your back and consider that a cat will eventually breathe that very same breath—those same molecules of air—tomorrow or next century.

The breath is so linked to our movements in a cat–cow flow. It is the tool that brings us from predator to prey and back again. "To be inspired is to be breathed upon," wrote Lyanda Lynn Haupt. Forget inspired; be instead, as she suggests, inspirable.[34] Instead of only flexing and arching the spine, experiment with side stretches and subtle twists. If you experience wrist pain at any time, take a break from the pose. Play in this space of movement-meets-breath for a minute or so, then sit comfortably and breathe in stillness for another minute or more.

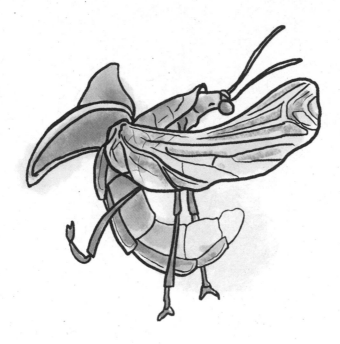

Chapter 5

TITTIBHA—FIREFLY

Fireflies are beyond-human being haiku. Instantaneous joy, and then it's gone. Off and on. A few short lines. A flash of light above ground after glowing eggs hatch and glowing larvae hunt beneath the earth or sometimes underwater.[1] Beetles with six legs live for fewer than six weeks. A single, mindful moment glimmers, then dims. It doesn't last.

❋ ❋ ❋

Fireflies are memories. Of searching for four-leaf clovers, barefoot in the cool grass, and finding none before the porch lights come on. Of a weathered picnic table next to a cabin before the coals in the grill are kissed with flame above which marshmallows hover and swirl. Of a photographer and his camera, flash off in the shrubfields while dusk falls, awaiting nature's night light. Of summers in West Virginia where the air burns with the love of family, both alive and already gone—some never known but born and buried in these hills with twinkling halos that are the home in my heart. So much searching, so much attention to light that pierces through almost-dark skies.

❋ ❋ ❋

Fireflies are flickering, unpredictable (to us) lanterns that depend on our discretion. At dusk, males of the most common firefly species in North America fly around at the perfect height from the ground to be caught by young and curious human hands. They illuminate in swooping motions creating momentary, glowing arcs.[2] Females waiting on the ground flash in response, revealing their locations so breeding may commence. Other species have their own nuanced flash codes, including those who glow in synchrony in Southeast Asia and the Great Smoky Mountains.[3] The most seemingly unobtrusive light pollution, the glow codes of flashlights or streetlamps, can disrupt firefly flickers for hours and therefore negatively impact reproduction and future firefly populations.[4]

❄ ❄ ❄

Fireflies, also called lightning bugs, are calendars marking the seasonal shift from spring to fall. They also mark the passing of years, secondhand memories, the transition from a little girl taking the lightning (specialized abdominal tissue[5]) from the "bug" (not "true bugs" in the taxonomic sense of the word). She goes from plucking glowing abdomens to wear as rings with her sister to cringing at confessing such cruelty.

❄ ❄ ❄

Fireflies are fireworks. Nothing good happens after dark, the saying goes, but what about twilight, that in-between time when insects attract and seduce? Some in earnest, to mate, and others to deceive and prey upon unsuspecting "bugs" with barely differently blinking butts. Some females use the codes of other species to trick and eat them, first flashing to mate and then blinking in different patterns to hunt males of multiple other species on the ground and on the wing, participating in a behavior called aggressive mimicry.[6] At dusk, there is just enough daylight left for the males to practice *viveka*, the yogic concept of discriminative discernment, to decide if the approaching female is a potential mate or trying to make a meal of him.[7] Survival is in the details.

❄ ❄ ❄

At 8:47 p.m. in early July, I watch the fireflies in a stand of trees in my neighborhood after returning from the grocery store. I turn off my headlights. Some flashes are high, and some are low, and I guess at the biological sex of my beetle neighbors on the wing. There is indeed movement to the glowing. One flashes a handful of times about nine feet above the ground. An outlier. A tall flier.

* * *

I contemplate how, sometimes, knowing the science behind the species changes our perceptions of the animals whose behavior we observe. Watching fireflies goes from being whimsical and fun to . . . well, a little stressful. Still, I pity the people whose summer evenings are not punctuated with beetle-breeding light displays. At a recent conference, I caught a firefly in my hand to give a couple of colleagues from Washington State their first up-close look at the little critter that resembles a winged sunflower seed with long black antennae and orange spots on his head. The humans' eyes and the beetle's abdomen lit up in synchrony.

* * *

Fireflies are *tittibha* in Sanskrit and in yoga studios where the air sparkles with enlightenment. Or is it the pageantry of tricks, mimicry, and occasional cannibalism?[8] Wrists root down bearing weight, thoraxes arch, hamstrings stretch, and feet take flight shimmering like wings, fragile and translucent underneath protective wing casings called elytra. The pose can improve balance, strengthen arms and hamstrings, and open the hips,[9] but are these benefits only in body or also in mind?

* * *

In *tittibhasana* I am a mere flicker. The "complex, interdependent system of behavioral mimicry"[10] that characterizes firefly reproduction is as challenging as the form of tittibhasana. Both require impressive feats of enlightened flight. And yet, most of the work of becoming firefly happens underground in the larval stage, unseen, a human working toward the asana. I strengthen my wrists, quadriceps, and core; practice hip-opening poses; and stretch out my hamstrings. I use blocks under my palms and the wall behind my hips for support as my body takes the shape of the firefly in intermittent waves of light. Inspiration glowing, I lift one foot, then place it back on the floor. Ignite, extinguish. It doesn't last.

* * *

Practice

LEAVE ONLY POETRY

You've likely heard the phrase, "Take only pictures, leave only footprints," and you may be familiar with its suggestion to minimize our impact on the environment. Now, even taking pictures has the potential to risk our own well-being, and that of other animals, in search of the "perfect" selfie to post on social media.

Processing my own encounters with wildlife through words has been deeply inspirational, providing a unique source of connection. In fact, this chapter began as a poem. When we "Leave Only Poetry," we write about our encounters with wildlife instead of always needing to document them with photographs. To give it a try, instead of taking a picture of the next animal you encounter, jot down a few words, a poem, or a description. Share that on social media, instead of a photograph. Use the hashtag #leaveonlypoetry. Reflect on the nature of your encounters as you write about them instead of capturing them in a picture. Are they more meaningful? Are you more mindful? Are you free to better appreciate sharing this planet with other beings when the stressful expectation to snap the perfect social media photo is absent?

The goal is to write, to enjoy writing, to share our words with others, and to add layers of meaning to our experiences with wildlife. If writing isn't your thing, speak your poetry aloud and enjoy the thrill of the impermanent nature of creative thought. I realize that not everyone considers themselves a poet. That's okay! A few adjectives strung together to remember a crow sighting in autumn, or the sound of a frog's voice, is poetry. "Leave Only Poetry" encourages writing as varied in quality and form as our encounters with other creatures can be. Sometimes, in an intimate yet annoying interaction, an animal sucks your blood. Sometimes you barely catch the blurry glimpse of a bear butt on the distant horizon. What is "good" poetry, anyway? Did it come from your heart? Is it an authentic response to your lived experience of the world? If so, I can't wait to read it! Here are some ideas to get you started:

- Think of words—any words—to describe the animal you observe. *White, feathery, graceful, boat, romance, intimidating, dinosaur.* List them. Rearrange them. Combine adjectives and nouns.

- Give the animal a new name. *Snowy giraffe bird.* It can be silly. It can be "stupid." But it's a new way of thinking.

- Write a "found poem" using a description of the animal in a field guide. What, that has already been written, resonates with you and your experience? It doesn't have to be a field guide. It can be a children's book. Or another poem. Or a comment made by your animal-observing companion.

- Imagine what the animal is thinking or feeling and put the text in quotations. Anthropomorphize away!

- Write a simile. Make a comparison. You could do it in fourth-grade language arts class, so you can do it now.

- Write a haiku. Forget 5-7-5! Three lines. Capture the moment. Just be you.

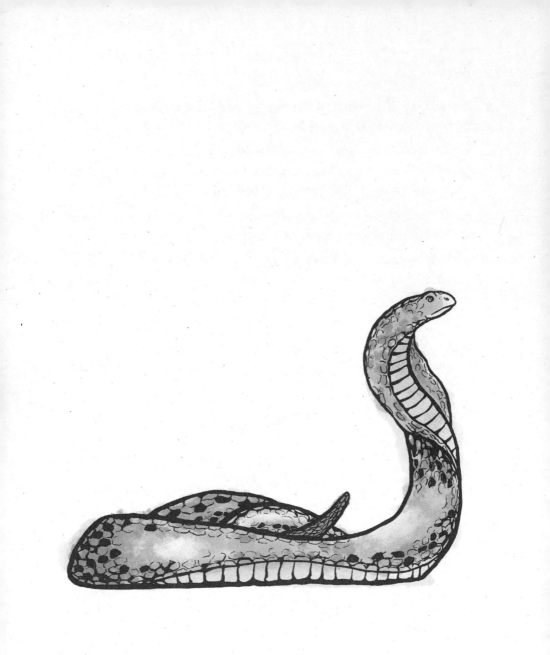

Chapter 6
BHUJANGA—SERPENT

I wish I could have written this chapter in a squiggle or a spiral instead of in straight rows of letters along a predetermined and never-changing path. Snakes coil. We recoil at the sight of anything that might be dangerous. Yet, the prefix *re-* implies that we were once also coiled like the serpent. We still are. In fact, I hope your body and mind coil, uncoil, and recoil intuitively as you read. . . .

Dennis Covington, author of *Salvation on Sand Mountain: Snake Handling and Redemption in Southern Appalachia*, wrote, "Feeling after God is dangerous business. . . ."[1]

Dangerous for whom, exactly?

Years ago, Covington's remarkable book introduced me to one of the most intriguing human–animal relationships I've ever explored. In short, believers "take up serpents," drink deadly substances, speak in tongues, and follow other signs from Mark 16:17–18. Those who are "right by God" survive bites from venomous snakes and sips of strychnine. This negative perception of snakes, while lesser known, exemplifies the general symbolism of serpents in the Christian tradition.

According to Pastor Andrew Hamblin, snakes are "death in your hand."[2] But how can something as spectacular and alive as a rattlesnake also be death?

The venomous snakes used for handling in these church services might include rattlesnakes, cottonmouths, copperheads, and cobras purchased via the exotic pet trade, or native species caught in the wild. The conditions in which they are kept for this purpose vary greatly. Snake experts at the Kentucky Reptile Zoo believe that the animals in the care of some of the snake-handling pastors lack appropriate treatment to behave as healthy snakes should. Their venom is likely weaker, they are less motivated to strike, and they live a fraction of their potential lifespans in these captive scenarios due to improper care. Another expert from the University of Georgia, Whitfield Gibbons, thinks that most snakes that become used to being handled are less likely to bite, so the religion of the handler doesn't matter.[3]

Although the anthropologist in me is curious to attend a signs-following service, there is something no visit to a church could answer: What is the experience like for the snake? Is the animal only a tool used to facilitate a human connection with the divine that excludes other creatures, or do serpents also experience God? Does divinity discriminate between human and snake? Between the species *sapiens* (wise) and *horridus* (horrible)?

❊ ❊ ❊

It's a Tuesday afternoon in the woodlands, but the timber rattlesnake doesn't know that. She distinguishes day from night, of course, but not Friday from Saturday. She's sunning herself on a rocky outcrop, not far from her den, still digesting a meal of juicy shrew from the previous morning. If snakes feel happiness, she is happy. If snakes feel God—or are God—she is divine.

Footsteps approach and shake the ground she suns on. It's something big, about the weight of a deer or a small bear. Instead of one furry mammal with four legs, it is two hairless mammals with two legs each. She notices that they stop traveling when they spot her. They sound and move differently from the quadrupedal animals she encounters more frequently. As the people inch closer she rattles her tail in polite admonishment before striking once at a long, metal pole with a hook on the end, which is extended toward her. Then she is wrangled into a bucket.

She spends the night inside a box with wooden sides and a clear, hinged lid that she shares with three other snakes. They are listless and lethargic. If snakes feel hope, these other rattlers have none left. There is neither light from the moon nor the quiet footsteps of foxes. Her chin rests on treated wood that is smooth and hard instead of the flaky softness of the fallen logs that cradle her head in the forest.

Toward the end of the next day, the box begins to move in rhythm with footsteps. A thump is followed by rumbles in a dark cave. She senses motion. Then, stillness and light again. There is more movement and the faint warmth of mammal hands that she senses with the pit organs on her face, through the walls of the box.

There is talking and singing. There are footsteps and hand claps. The box lid opens.

"Careful with that one," someone says, "we caught her just yesterday." What is a warning to the human animal is a series of vibrations to the snake.

Cool tongs clamp down firmly on either side of her body, not far behind her head, as she is lifted from the box. A breeze blows through the open door at the back of the building.

A man sings and shouts and dances, thrusting her skyward. Occasionally, he yells at her as if she is the devil herself, born in the nearby woods, an unwelcome neighbor as horrid as her Latin species name suggests—or more so.

The vibrations and strange scents crescendo. If snakes feel fear, she is scared. Her rattle has no use now. Warm mammal hands prevent her from coiling tightly into a pile of comforting curves as she would if threatened on the ground. Her fangs are folded against the roof of her mouth, her venom glands full.

A day ago, she was basking in the divine light of the forest. Tonight, serpents taken up, it is the signs-followers' turn to feel God.

She does not strike.

✳ ✳ ✳

"Is she poisonous?"

I've been asked this question countless times, by children and adults on guided hikes, upon finding an eastern ratsnake sunning near a rock wall. What they mean, of course, is, "Should I fear her?" or "Can she hurt me?" What they also mean is, "Is she venomous?" To be harmed by a *venomous* snake you must first be bitten by them, and the snake must inject their venom into your body. Alternatively, to be harmed by a *poisonous* snake you would have to ingest the animal (and be small enough for the poison to affect you, which you likely are not). There are only a couple kinds of poisonous snakes in the world: the keelbacks, and the garters, who live in

North America and become poisonous through their diet of toxic newts. Still, the answer is, "No, she can't hurt you." Unless you are a newt.

Venomous snakes instill so much fear. Yes, *they* could hurt you, and in some places venomous snakes are an all-too-frequent cause of death. By one estimate, as many as 100,000 people die each year of venomous snakebites worldwide.[4] Yet, most of our "encounters" with snakes are perceived only by the snake.

I encountered a venomous snake years ago. I was biking with my dad at Flatwoods Park north of Tampa, and we decided to explore a sandy trail through the scrub habitat in the center of a paved loop. Halfway through our ride, we came across a couple stopped in the trail, staring at an eastern diamondback rattlesnake right in the middle of the path. The couple turned around and biked out from the direction they came. The snake was stretched out in the sun, his well-camouflaged body only slightly curved. He barely moved as we approached with caution, but he did rattle, an audible signal for what our eyes already noticed. The grasses and saw palmettos were tall and thick on both sides of the trail, so it was a tight squeeze for human and bike to pass outside of striking range of the rattler. We also wondered whether he was digesting a meal, as we observed a particularly bulbous section of the snake's body. My dad managed to get around the snake's tail end as he slowly moved from the trail into the vegetation, but I was paralyzed with fear. The only thing that got me moving was my dad threatening to pedal off without me.

"Well, I wouldn't really have left you behind!" he said recently, laughing as he recalled the incident.

I remember listening to cedar flute music in my car after this bike ride and bristling at the sound of a rattle instrument. But once the fear wore off, I was able to appreciate the extraordinary function of this magical, musical tail. A generous warning. With awe and respect, I realized that the snake had communicated with me to avoid a situation that would have been more stressful for us both. Cobras are equally polite. They lift their heads and spread their hoods as if to suggest, "Hey, do you see me? I am right here. Please mind the serpent." Instead of coiling and rattling so that we might hear them, cobras arise and appear larger so that we might see them. The hood is a gentle admonition.

Hooded serpents are significant in multiple religions. They even protect the gods. A cobra with multiple hoods sheltered the Buddha from the
elements as he achieved enlightenment.[5] It makes me wonder: What was
in it for the cobras if the Buddha became awakened? What motivated their
care and attention to the scale-less, four-limbed mammal sitting so still
underneath the Bodhi tree? As it turns out, the Buddha repaid the snakes
by teaching nonviolence toward and compassion for all creatures. He knew
that he was once a snake. While one religious perspective of the serpent
conjures fear and punishment, another offers protection and devotion to
spiritual practice.

The deceptively simple *bhujangasana*, commonly referred to as cobra
pose, can be as misunderstood by yoga practitioners as snakes are by people
across the world. In fact, *bhujanga* means "snake" or "serpent," not "cobra"
specifically, though the pose does mimic the raised hood of the cobra as the
body lies prone, belly to the earth. Pressing palms into that same earth,
the torso rises; head, shoulders, and chest open forward, a simultaneous
grounding and uplifting.

Bhujangasana is a backbend felt mostly in the middle of the spine.
The pose has the potential to strengthen the back muscles, open the chest,
improve flexibility and alignment of the spine, and act as a "great antidote
to lots of sitting."[6] In it, our eyes point downward (unlike snakes) and that's
exactly where we should fix our gaze in order to protect the backs of our
necks.[7] Like the cobra, the muscles in our back and torso allow us to lift our
body from the earth. In this pose, we are reminded how our yoga practice
encourages a sensory experience of the subtleties of the body and its environment, much like a snake who reads vibrations and smells with a forked
tongue.[8]

When I teach nature yoga to children, we embody a different kind of
serpent. The eastern hognose is a nonvenomous snake native to my home
habitat in the Mid-Atlantic. These native snakes are adorable with their little
pig snouts and dramatic displays when threatened. The kids and I practice
an armless bhujangasana, but on the count of three we all roll over and
thrash around, playing dead like the hognose. We writhe, belly up, with our
tongues hanging out. Kids love it!

In *Light on Yoga*, a comprehensive text that describes over two hundred asanas, B.K.S. Iyengar references another version of the pose. In it, the arms reach back and bind above the knees, making the backbend much more intense while also making the pose look a lot more like an armless cobra with a raised hood, "like a serpent about to strike."[9] This variation is not accessible to me or to most of my students. While teaching bhujangasana I am known to say, "Snakes don't have arms" and we practice an armless version without a bind, using the back muscles and opening through the chest to rise without straining the back.[10] It is a more subtle expression of the pose, yes, but one with more anatomical integrity. Snakes don't have legs either, but our limbs are what ground us as we press down into the floor to rise up.[11] An armless cobra inches us slightly closer to what it might feel like to be a snake, while using the arms allows us to embody the physical shape of the cobra. If nothing else, the next time you practice bhujangasana, I hope a hooded serpent slithers for a second through the uneven ground of your conscious mind.

✳ ✳ ✳

On one of the first few handfuls of autumn nights when the temperature dipped below freezing in the eastern panhandle of West Virginia, I visited the nature center at Cool Spring Preserve. It was pitch black when I entered with my friend and former colleague, Amy Moore. After flicking on the lights, we headed downstairs past walls plastered with cartoon bird decals to where the animals lived. There, the aquatic turtles, Louie the river cooter and Poppie the red-eared slider, swam frantically and clawed against the panes of their glass tanks, hoping for a late-night snack. We walked up to Scute the box turtle, whose eyes were still closed as he nestled into his little log dome for a night of slumber. Willow the wood turtle couldn't be bothered to greet us. I love all these turtles, but it was the newest resident education animal that I came to meet that night.

Esther the corn snake arrived at the Potomac Valley Audubon Society in August 2021. Amy, the organization's lead educator and naturalist, explained that Esther was confiscated by the state from someone selling snakes into the illegal pet trade. While it is unlawful to possess native reptiles without the proper permits, it was also impossible to release Esther after she spent time in captivity due to the risk of disease transmission to wild reptiles. So, she became an animal ambassador with whom Amy and her team would work to educate visitors about native wildlife.

"We hope that Esther will help dispel fears or misconceptions about snakes among our program participants. Ultimately, we want to inspire love and appreciation for the wild animals that these ambassadors represent," she explained.[12]

"Why did you name her Esther?"

"Try saying it like this: Esssther." Amy grinned.

Esssther was napping beneath a layer of wood chips, but Amy carefully pulled her out and placed her in my hands. Waking right up, Esther seemed to appreciate the warmth my skin provided. She became more active as the minutes passed, her body undulating between my fingers and around angled elbow creases. I marveled at how a creature could be so soft but not furry. She was an earthy tan color with striking tangerine splotches that matched my henna-stained fingernails. Her spots were outlined in black, and her body curled perfectly into the contours of my hands as her head dipped in and out of my jacket pocket. With big, dark pupils and a rounded snout, Esther was the cutest snake I'd ever met. Her coral-colored tongue tickled my skin.

Corn snakes are native to the east coast of the U.S. from the south to the mid-Atlantic. They hunt for rodents in open fields and seek shelter in underground burrows in adjacent forests.[13] Unfortunately, Esther's wild kin are commonly mistaken for copperheads and therefore killed. Many of the aforementioned hognose snakes meet their death at the chop of a shovel for the same reason. Their cobra-like hoods don't help, but their adorable, smooshed snoots should! The point is not even that we shouldn't kill non-venomous snakes because they aren't copperheads . . . the point is that only a small fraction of venomous snakes harm people at all. Snake expert and advocate Dr. David Steen explains it like this: "Look, a snake isn't being aggressive just because it does something other than roll over and die when approached with a shovel. A scared snake will try to defend itself, just as you would." Snakes aren't looking for a fight. In fact, one study in South

Carolina found that students searching for captive pythons in a "large out-door enclosure" only had a 1 percent chance of actually seeing one.[14] So, while you may be looking for snakes, they would rather you not find them.

In a 2020 *New York Times* article titled "How My Pet Snake Taught Me to Really See," Paul McAdory wrote, "The snake is as much symbol as animal, and this oversaturation of meaning prevents us from seeing the snake clearly."[15] This is brilliant. From fertility to death, protection to deception, from demons to the divine, serpents simultaneously represent the best and worst of our human relationships with wildlife and nature. But what does all this have to do with the animals who live on the planet with us this very moment? When we rely too heavily on symbols, we are distanced from the beings in front of us. This disconnect from nature leads to the "evil-ing" of an adorable Esssther or the vilification of beyond-human beings because they use venom to defend and feed themselves.

Making snakes into symbols of the devil is why the snake-handling component of worship in signs-following churches is, in my opinion, prob-lematic. Not only does this symbolism imply that they are not worthy of humane treatment, but in this context, the snake in hand may indeed feel fear only because who they are as an individual is inconsistent with what they symbolize to the human holding them. In conducting research for this book, it occurred to me how snakes seem to be treated more harshly in places where snakebite deaths are less frequent and access to healthcare in case of bites is more widely available. In contrast, in parts of the world where deaths do occur, the snakes are often still viewed as sacred, proving that we can protect ourselves and our families' safety without uncondi-tional intolerance for an entire taxon of creatures.

So, is seeking God dangerous business? It is if we find the sacred in places and within beings where the established religious institutions don't want us to find God. To see divinity instead of the devil in the serpent. For some, mindfully encountering and embodying other creatures may indeed be dangerous—not for us as individuals, but for the dominant systems in place. In our Western patriarchal society, if we understand that we are bhu-janga we may be less likely to blindly follow the existing human systems of oppression and inequality, the same systems that claim dominion and control over nature for profit and convenience. For example, embodying a cow is threatening to the factory farming industry, and embodying a mountain is problematic for the coal companies who blow summits to smithereens for unsustainable sources of energy at the expense of so many lives.

Connecting with animals can help other humans too. These practices are dangerous, in the best possible way, for those who wish to perpetuate the idea that certain beings are more powerful due to the color of their skin, the privilege with which they were born, or the "species" category into which they fall in this lifetime. Let us shed that nonsense with every inch of our serpentine spines. Snakeskins from different species, discarded and inside out, are remarkably similar in color and pattern once they are shed. Let's lift our torsos from the earth and spread our hoods to protect all oppressed animals, limbed or not, and their exploited ecosystems. And let us not forget that acknowledging our Yoga—our unity—is never meant to downplay the suffering of others or to ignore our differences. Realizing that "we are all one" means that we work to address the foundational and systemic causes of others' suffering because that suffering is also our own.

We placed Esther on the cool, concrete floor of the nature center that night, only for a moment, to watch her move without the restraint of hands. She flowed like a river viewed from the window of an airplane. As sacred as being with a snake can feel, I tried to stay present, appreciating Esther as an individual instead of a symbol for something—anything—else. We returned her to her bed of wood chips.

I am grateful for the occasional opportunity to hold a snake. Serpent bodies are so assured, so solid and confident in your hands. They move with such precision and ease that I wished, on a dark November night, that I was cold-blooded and covered in scales myself. I guess I'm a bit of a snake handler after all. As I "took up a serpent" who was loved by some and vilified by others, I thanked Esther for the small role she plays in the "un-deviling" of snakes in Appalachia, one friendly encounter at a time. Or not. Sometimes a snake is just a snake, and that is enough.

Esssther is always enough.

✳ ✳ ✳

Practice

"SUFI GRIND" KRIYA

A chapter chock-full of yoga and snakes would be incomplete without a mention of *kundalini,* a Sanskrit term translated as "having a coil."[16] It is also defined as energy or a serpent "coiled at the base of our spine, embodying our primal survival instincts, which can rise up and stir the flowering wisdom in our mind."[17] Certain kriyas (sets of practices or actions to achieve a certain outcome)[18] are designed to awaken this coiled serpent energy at the base of the spine.

Waking snakes are slightly anxiety producing, but I take inspiration from the serpents themselves. I have been honored, on multiple early spring days, to watch as dozens of eastern ratsnakes emerged from their winter hibernaculum located in a culvert under a gravel road. I installed "brake for snakes" signs so drivers would yield to awakening serpents. When they rouse, they are beautiful and mysterious and you want to watch them move, to see what they are capable of; but, you are careful too. Respectfully cautious. You yield to rattles (not of ratsnakes, but other species) and rumblings of what is inappropriate for your own body and mind. Every fall the snakes retreat underground again.

To give a kriya called the "sufi grind" a try, sit on the ground in a comfortable cross-legged position or in a chair. Move your torso in a clockwise circle, imagining that the movement originates from your hips. Let your hands be loose on your knees, as if you don't need them. Let your chin hinge gently forward as you move forward and as you move backward. Inhale forward, exhale back. Unite movement and breath. The speed at which you move is up to you. Don't overthink it. Be serpentine. Rotate this way for a minute or two, and then reverse directions for an equal amount of time.[19] Treat it like a dance or a trance, a simple warm-up for the spine, or an acknowledgment of the snake within. When your body stills, sit for a silent moment and observe the effect of the kriya on your body and mind. A Tamil proverb says, "Only a snake knows the leg of another snake."[20] There is only one way to know what it's like to be a snake: you must become a snake. We needn't fear returning to the state of our original coiling. It is where we have infinite potential.

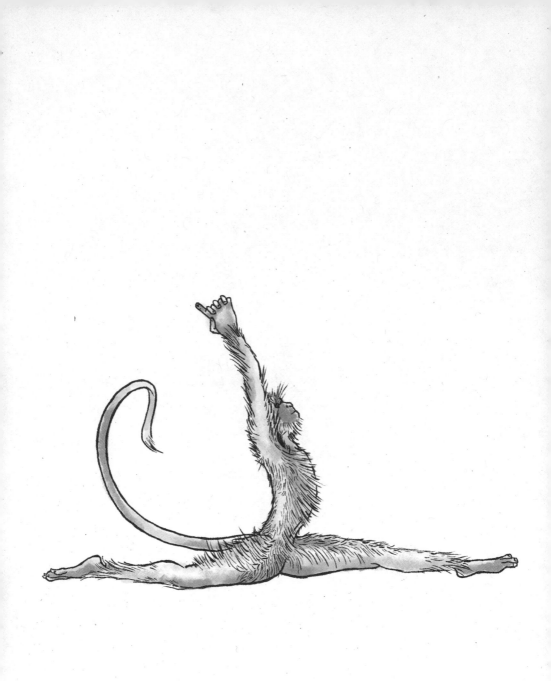

Chapter 7
HANUMAN—MONKEY

Monkey mind is a term used by Buddhists and others in the meditation community to refer to the tendencies of our distracted minds to wander. The analogy is that we jump from one thought to the next like monkeys leaping mindlessly through the branches, chattering aloud as they travel through the forest canopy. The term *monkey mind* has a negative connotation, and this bothers me. I would argue that monkeys are far more mindful than most humans, living in the present more often than we do. We are especially busy and anxious animals, either dwelling in the past or planning for the future. Or both. At the same time. While checking our smartphones. Apparently, we are supposed to harness the monkey mind, but why would we want to "tame" ourselves in this way? We do not have to spend much time observing primates to realize that they have agency. All my encounters with monkeys are more meaningful when they are allowed to be their "wild" selves, existing in the world in their habitats and homes on their own terms.

Yes, as the analogy suggests, monkeys travel through the trees—with a purpose. Above motorcycles winding along roads through the forest, the moor macaque monkeys I used to study leave their natal social groups behind to join new ones and begin breeding. Juveniles play with each other and learn important life skills. Troops head toward certain fig trees, mouths salivating at memories of especially ripe and juicy fruits. They expand their home ranges to include better resources or to compensate for anthropogenic disturbances like large- or small-scale deforestation or development. They travel to grow up, reproduce, forage, and avoid danger.

Monkey movement also sets into motion other important processes that connect them to us and to the ecological systems of which they are a part. As they travel, they flush insects from the forest canopy that are then eaten by birds who flit around awaiting an easy meal. Because they typically move around in large and conspicuous groups, monkeys alert other animals to the location of available food and potential predators. Many species disperse seeds as they poop in different places, ensuring future generations of forest resources for their descendants and ours. They influence landscapes and the lives of plants and other animals in their own habitats and beyond. Monkeys on the move quite literally change the world.

Monkey "chatter" communicates crucial information like desires, emotions, warnings, and past experiences. Vervet monkeys, for example, are famous for their alarm calls, which vary to indicate different types of threats. The vocalizations they emit for feline, avian, and reptilian predators all sound different to suggest how the group of monkeys should react. To avoid a terrestrial cat, the monkeys are safer to run up into the branches of a tree, but to escape an eagle in flight they move down into thicker vegetation.[1] They also communicate about each other, including their status in (or out of) the group and individuals' positions in dominance hierarchies. Vervets can even use these alarm calls to manipulate others, for example by "lying" about a leopard nearby to disrupt a fight with a neighboring group, or by deceiving others about the presence of an eagle to encourage them to leave a food source.[2] Campbell monkeys, a species of guenon also from Africa, use calls to indicate the immediacy of a threat and whether or not they heard or saw the predator, making clear the difference between "Careful . . . it's nearby" and "Hide! It's here!"[3] Monkeys communicate to avoid predators, maintain social groups, prevent aggression, and aid in reconciliation. These are no trivial issues in the life of a primate, human or beyond-human. Chatter matters.

Even if monkeys do occasionally dilly-dally, staring for a whimsical moment at a caterpillar marching along a stem or watching a rushing waterfall navigate the rocks—isn't that mindfulness too? Primatologist Barbara Smuts once wrote about an observation she made of a "baboon sangha."[4] The term *sangha* typically refers to a Buddhist monastic community, but the baboon version involved the entire social group sitting in still and quiet contemplation around reflective pools of water.[5] Shouldn't we strive to live more like the monkeys, one minute crashing through the branches on a quest for a nourishing snack and the next being groomed by a friend in a sleepy state of relaxed ecstasy?

I wish there were a better term, one more informed about monkeys, to refer to our own powerful minds. But I can also see why monkey mind resonates. We relate to our fellow primates as we struggle to exist mindfully in the world. We all share primate minds that are at times distracted and full of chatter, but also immensely capable of connection, compassion, calm, and awe. If we delve a little deeper into primate behavior and cognition, we might consider ourselves lucky to have a monkey mind!

※ ※ ※

While I no longer use my own primate mind to study living monkeys, they did lead me to Hanuman the monkey god. He is the reason I was drawn to the Ramayana, the ancient story about Rama and Sita, a royal couple who, together, represent the divine masculine and feminine incarnate. They are forced apart, full of despair, by Ravana, the "villain" who represents our own struggles to reunite with the divine. Ravana captures Sita and imprisons her on the island of Lanka. Thanks to the help of Hanuman, Rama and Sita are eventually reunited. This story of separation and unification happens again and again, throughout the story, throughout our lives, and throughout time. Not only does the Ramayana come from the same rich, cultural tradition as yoga and its associated practices in South Asia, but the story is literally about Yoga, the union of the divine masculine and feminine. Whether we practice asana, meditation, service to our community, or all of the above, yoga is the practice we use to unite the Rama and Sita within us, to yoke together the divine human and beyond-human, with Hanuman as our monkey-minded guide.

Throughout the story, Sita, who was born from a furrow in the earth, demonstrates affection for nature and monkeys in particular. Like Sita, I adore Hanuman, the hero of the entire epic, who represents strength, vitality, energy, faith, courage, intelligence, and eternal youth.[6] While devotees of Hanuman are unlikely to stress over which extant primate species he represents, some anthropologists regard the question with interest. In the human primate community, there is disagreement on the subject. Most people think he is either representative of a macaque or a langur, both Asian monkeys; the former more terrestrial and omnivorous, and the latter more arboreal and herbivorous. He has red fur according to some sources and golden fur according to others.[7] Neither macaques nor langurs have red fur, except for the maroon langur of Borneo and its nearby islands. The bulb of longer hair at the end of Hanuman's tail suggests lion-tailed macaque, an endangered species from southern India.

I may be biased, but Hanuman looks more macaque- than langur-like to me, especially his facial features. In the South Asian depiction with which I am most familiar, he has kind eyes, a protruding jaw, and well-defined muscles. He wears gold and jewels and is draped in fancy cloth. Southeast Asian versions of Hanuman vary in appearance from the Indian depictions, just as the Ramayana itself changes as the stories are shared over time and spread into new areas. At the temple in the famed Ubud Monkey Forest in Bali, a carved stone Hanuman statue wears a menacing expression on his dragon-like face and carries an oversized mace, ready to strike. He is more fierce than friendly. We can only assume that Hanuman is linked to multiple existing species, depending on interpretation and primate distribution, across his devotees' geographic range.

In behavior, macaques and langurs are both similar to the monkeys of the Ramayana, called *vanaras*, whose antics would shock no primatologist. It is fascinating to trace through the texts how the tellers and retellers of these stories were such astute observers of primate behavior. Vali, a powerful monkey king in the epic, operates within a social hierarchy in which dominant males mate with females and receive preference while foraging.[8] The vanaras tease sages in meditation and playfully steal their possessions, forage in orchards, and gorge themselves on honey. Yes, even the primates of the Ramayana do some monkeying around, but it's all for a purpose. What makes Hanuman so special is that he represents what stands in direct opposition to the concept of monkey mind. He is a monkey whose mind is focused on a single task that he performs out of devotion to the ones he loves. He is the quintessential monkey.

So, if Hanuman is a god capable of flying great distances, eating the sun, and carrying medicinal mountains to heal wounded warriors (not to mention an admirable super-devotion to God), what does that have to do with monkeys alive today? Do these distinctions and comparisons to extant species matter? One anthropologist wrote that it is unclear, when Hanuman was first conceptualized, how people distinguished between multiple species,[9] and if I have learned one thing from my own anthropological studies it is that there are more ways of knowing animals than Western science acknowledges or allows for. What it boils down to is generally good news for Asian primates in areas where Hinduism is widely practiced. In India, depending on the location and many diverse interpretations of the Ramayana, any primate species may be eligible for (somewhat conditional) sacred status on the subcontinent.[10] Many scholars agree that Hanuman worship grew out of devotion to *yakshas,* nature spirits who guarded the earth.[11]

Now, to many Hindus, the monkeys found at temples throughout India are living representatives of the Ramayana hero, and feeding them ensures blessings and protection from the gods. The monkeys receive more food on the worship days associated with Hanuman, Tuesdays and Saturdays, and on festival days or other celebrations. In one sense, these temples are places where earthly animals and their divine forms seamlessly coexist. In another sense, it is chaos. As my mother-in-law said of Indian monkey temples, "Here, we don't need to give the monkeys *prasaad* [a ritual food offering]. They just take it!" The feedings resemble less of a consensual, spiritual exchange and more of an intense display of social group dynamics exacerbated by the presence of people and food. There may be a lot more snatching and screaming involved than your typical religious offering!

Some people believe that Hanuman is present until the day people no longer recite the Ramayana. During his time here on earth, what better form for him to take than Asia's lively and clever primates? Hanuman travels from the land of the monkeys, not only across oceans and skies, from mountains to islands, but also from the things we know are not two, but one: from animal to God, from heaven to earth, from separate self to Universal Self.

As I search for Hanuman within myself and the world around me, I wonder: Is my sense that monkeys have always been sacred what drew me to Hanuman? Or did my deepening personal relationship with Hanuman inspire me to see the monkeys I used to see through a scholarly lens through a spiritual lens instead? My introduction to Hanuman's grace was through monkeys and my encounters with monkeys are infused with Hanuman's grace. People (including my understandably Rama-critical mother-in-law) ask me why I love Hanuman so much, and I sputter a useless answer. It feels a lot like someone asking, "Why do you love animals so much?" I don't know, but it is one of my truest truths.

All the monkeys I've ever encountered are Hanuman. He was there when I encountered my first wild primate, a long-tailed macaque we called Susu (Malay for "sweet milk"), on top of Mount Santubong. He greeted me on my Himalayan honeymoon when langurs materialized around us as we trekked down the mountain, and he was there among the sand and the mangroves and the proboscis monkeys. He was in the moor macaques whose fuzzy butts fled my approach in the Sulawesi forests. And he is there every time I visit the Silver River, watching the water flow with the rhesus macaques whether I detect their presence or not. With gods and with monkeys, they can sense us better than we can sense them. But that doesn't stop me from seeking.

I love to visit Hanuman temples whenever I visit Asia, but I also experience the nagging feeling that my expressions of devotion within these physical spaces feel performative. My personal acts of worship do not occur within the ornately carved stone walls of temples to the sound of bells and *bhajans* ("devotional songs"). They happen when I chant the forty verses of praise called the Hanuman Chalisa in my car in the middle of traffic. They happen when I experience turbulence during air travel and imagine Hanuman beneath the plane, holding it up with all the effortlessness and compassion with which he carried the mountain with the healing herb to the battlefield.

I once visited a hilltop temple in Hyderabad with a fifty-foot-tall Hanuman. I circled the idol thrice, slipping on smooth, wet marble in my bare feet. I touched his giant toe and received his blessings. I marveled at his massive tail while pigeons perched on his bejeweled crown. I wear a Hanuman pendant around my neck and scatter idols of various sizes around our house. You can never have too many. Still, in desperate times I forget he's all around me. But the truth is: I am Hanuman. So are you. He doesn't fly into our hearts when we chant his name or when we light a stick of incense. He lives there, his own heart ripped wide open, ready to serve the divine. In fact, every beat of our primate heart is a reminder of that divinity inside us. The depth of my devotion is the same whether Hanuman is three stories tall or a bronze idol no taller than a grasshopper.

* * *

As with garudasana, *hanumanasana* is named not after a living animal, but after the deity who is half human, half animal. Some say that Hanuman is associated with asana because he invented the physical postures as he mimicked and embodied the other creatures of the forest.[12] Others believe he developed the popular yoga sequence, the sun salutation, to thank the Surya, the sun, for his teachings.[13] Similarly, Hanuman learned pranayama, breath control practices, from Vayu, his father the wind god. He then shared this knowledge with humans, which is why pranayama is one of the eight limbs of yoga today.[14] Hanuman is the perfect yogi because he is the embodiment of union. The pose that represents him is also referred to as "the full split," and is said to commemorate Hanuman's famous leap across the ocean from Lanka to the Himalayas to fetch the mountain with a medicinal plant and carry it back to Rama's wounded brother.[15]

Many years ago, I practiced the pose I now call hanumanasana in a bright blue leotard sparkling with silver sequins at the conclusion of a baton-twirling routine to the tune of "Cotton Eye Joe." I've been striving back toward the posture ever since. Separation and reunion. What we seek from Hanuman involves our body as well as our mind.[16] During hanumanasana, one leg stretches forward and the other back while my heart turns toward the front leg. Arms extend toward the sky or palms press together in front of my heart. Although close to the ground, I am flying. The pose requires a great deal of flexibility and strength in the hips and the backs of the legs.[17] It is a challenging pose, but one that can be practiced through many accessible variations. You can practice the split on your back with a strap or scarf looped around your raised foot. You can practice it while standing at a wall, or by placing blocks under your hips as I do. Upside-down or right-side-up, I am graceful in the pose, like I could also move mountains.

It is Hanuman's fearless faith and devotion that give him the confidence to accomplish difficult tasks such as leaping across an ocean[18] the way living monkeys leap across gaps in the forest canopy. The split, with legs reaching in opposite directions, is a unifying posture. It bridges, bringing two separate things together. The trick is that we *are* that to which we are devoted. Our monkey minds can help us recall our own divinity. But here's the best part: Hanuman forgets his divinity too. Although he is always praying for the strength and grace to achieve difficult things, he is fully capable of it all from the start.[19] How primate of him. And of us. So much forgetting and remembering. This is the practice. Hanuman is our guide. May you carry mountains of devotion always in your heart.

Practice
"UNTAMING THE MIND MONKEYS" MEDITATION

Sit in a comfy spot with your spine nice and long. Root down into your seat with the groundedness of the terrestrial monkeys—the baboons and the macaques whose feet and hands touch the earth. Breathe in the grace of mindful and mischievous arboreal monkeys the world over—the spider monkeys and howlers who spend most of their lives not in the trees but of them. Breathe out devotion to your own human primate self.

Meditate. Let your goal be an untaming of the mind. Be a primatologist of thought. Instead of watching your mind monkeys swing on by, try following them through the forest, respectfully observing them without judgment. As they groom and play and rest and move. Bring your binoculars. Stay in this meditation as long as it brings you closer to something positive, not further from it. Trust your monkey mind.

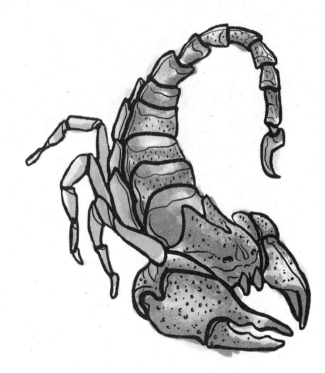

Chapter 8

VRSCHIKA—SCORPION

I once spent the night at an Iban longhouse. I was in college, studying abroad for the summer in Malaysian Borneo, on the ancestral lands of the Dayak people. The building was newly constructed with brick only six years prior, after a fire destroyed the previous structure made of wood and bamboo. The exterior was painted a cheerful shade of yellow. Front doors led into an enclosed porch with matching pillars and ornate blue-and-white tile that served as a common area for all twenty or so families who lived there. I was a part of the first group of tourists to ever visit this longhouse, a fact that made me feel an uncomfortable mixture of adventure, voyeurism, and despair.

Inhabitants bustled in and out of doors as they cooked for over five hours, preparing dinner for us all to share. I used a mortar and pestle to crush ginger and cassava leaves, entertaining the women who eventually took the heavy utensil from my hand to fix and finish my shabby attempt at helping in the kitchen. We ate fish, chicken, and pork cooked in tubes of hollow bamboo over hot coals in an old metal drum that was cut in half. For dessert, there were green oranges bursting with unexpected flavor.

After dinner and time for washing up, we sat together in the common area on woven mats drinking rice wine called *tuak*. Then we danced the Pucho Pucho. At first the choreography seemed almost identical to the electric slide, but then we added variations involving clapping, waving, disco pointing, and little kicks that brought *Seinfeld's* Elaine Benes to life in rural Malaysia. Later, we tried traditional Iban dancing with its slow and rhythmic moves, then lay down to sleep on mattresses on the living room floor.

An old woman came in, thin and wrinkled in the dim lighting, and cackled out loud at the sight of me and the other students lined up in a row.

As we left the longhouse the next morning, we noticed a seven-inch-long scorpion right outside the living room door. He was beaten to death with a shoe as we slept, someone explained. Never to strike again.

I wondered if the scorpion raised his tail to sting the rubber tread before the shoe crashed down upon him, or if this squished little soul simply paid the price for the harm another individual had wrought. In fact, the behavior so associated with this animal represents only a small fraction, a split second here and there, of the life of a scorpion's six years or more on earth.

The sting. It does often characterize the fearful encounters humans have with scorpions. The four-inch-long deathstalker scorpion has the fastest strike of all, clocking in at fifty-one inches per second.[1] Yet, scorpions do not have an inexhaustible source of venom; they need to rest up and replenish between strikes.[2] In addition to their stinger, scorpions also have pincers called pedipalps that they use to catch prey. Many scorpions attack with pedipalps first and only use venom if needed. Some studies found that scorpions use their stinger one-third of the time and only for larger prey.[3]

As much as we fear scorpions with their quick strikes and venomous stings, critters in the bee family kill ten times more people in the U.S. than all arachnids and snakes combined.[4] And people love bees! Imagine if, in addition to pollinator gardens, bee baths, and bee condos, we created little scorpion shelters and made dark corners available and appealing for prime spiderweb weaving. I picture trick-or-treating toddlers who ditch striped shirts and antennae headbands. Instead, they slip sugar-sticky hands into plush pedipalps and attach sharp, bulbous tails to their elastic-waisted pants.

The sting is less of an aggressive attack and more of a well-calculated and precisely executed decision on which the scorpion's survival may depend. Sometimes the strike of the venomous tail is used for hunting prey.[5] The sharp part of the stinger, called the aculeus, is like the tine of a fork that we use to impale a wedge of greasy skillet potato. The movement of the fork in our hand is quick and aggressive like an ambush-style attack. But we are hungry and fried potatoes are filling; they taste of garlic and salt and happiness, and we are enjoying an outdoor Sunday brunch with friends. Our use of forks to eat does not make us malicious.

Other times the scorpion's venomous tail is used for defense,[6] poised like keychain pepper spray in the hands of a woman pursued by an entitled and dangerous man. She never wants to use it, but she's glad she has it. Cradling the small canister in her palm, finger on the plastic trigger, she constantly recalculates risk as she moves down a dimly lit city sidewalk looking back over her shoulder. We've got scorpions all wrong.

The sting is misunderstood, and sometimes, so am I. I've been told that I'm too intense, that I have a negative edge, that I need to smile more so others think I'm "more approachable." Some days others' venom gets the best of me, but other times, like the critters who have evolved alongside scorpions for millennia, I too can survive substantial levels of toxicity. Grasshopper mice, for example, eat bark scorpions and can withstand up to twenty times the venom as an unfortunate lab mouse. In the Middle East, the fan-fingered gecko can survive the equivalent of one hundred stings from the yellow scorpion.[7] Christie Wilcox, author of *Venomous: How Earth's Deadliest Creatures Mastered Biochemistry*, wrote, "A spider or scorpion can be unceremoniously crushed under our feet, yet some of their venoms can take us out just as easily."[8] Can't you also relate? Sometimes life results in the annihilation of our emotional exoskeletons with an audible and unceremonious crunch. And sometimes, we defend ourselves, our values, our loved ones, and our homes with a seemingly infinite supply of potent and invincible venom.

Scorpions exhibit other behaviors that endear them to us if we take a mindful moment to inquire beyond the sting. For example, the courtship behavior of a scorpion pair includes the holding of pedipalps, a couple's stroll called a promenade (I desperately want to meet the romantic scientist who developed the scorpion courtship ethogram), and, for the kinkier of my dear readers, a sexual stinging delivered by the male to the female.[9] Sometimes they move back and forth, touching mouth parts while grasping each other.[10] I might dare to call that dancing and kissing. After all this foreplay, a spermatophore is deposited by the male and picked up by the female. *Ooh la la.* (See, it can be fun to anthropomorphize!)

Scorpion mothers are unique in the world of terrestrial invertebrates, giving live birth after a relatively long gestation period, then caring for their young until their first molt.[11] Mothers and scorplings (that's the endearing term for baby scorpions) learn to recognize each other using a combination of touch, sight, and chemical cues. This association is important to the vulnerable little scorplings who ride on their mother's back for protection from predators, access to better habitat, and hydration as the mother passes water through her body to her young.[12] Wouldn't many human parents love for their young to develop a protective exoskeleton before dispersing into the big, wide world?

※ ※ ※

Sam Sheikali (known online as "Saminal Planet") is a medical doctor and wildlife enthusiast with an interest in *envenomation*, the human body's exposure to toxins from venomous animals. The study of envenomation allows doctors to more effectively diagnose and treat bites and stings, even when the patient doesn't know what species was involved.

Right before our scheduled call Sam sent me a picture of a two-inch-long, chocolate-colored scorpion poised on the edge of his hand. A couple of days earlier he went outside, looked under a rock, and there she was. Apparently, if you go searching for scorpions at night, a black light will illuminate their glowing exoskeletons. This adaptation may have evolved to help scorpions sense ultraviolet light with their whole bodies so they can avoid it and stay better hidden during the night.[13]

Sam commuted to an overnight shift at the emergency room as we talked. When I asked why he was interested in venomous critters, he said, "That's the million-dollar question! I guess it's the power of it. This little thing has such an incredible, biochemical tool that helps them live their lives and defend themselves."

So, he is interested in the sting.

He continued, "When people see scorpions, they see this perceived scary thing that they think wants to hurt them, but they are so much more than that. Sure, they have their defense mechanisms—like humans, right? We're all just trying to survive. Scorpions do the same. If you're not messing with them, they won't mess with you."

He has done a little messing, although it was unintentional. Sam shared that he has been stung twice by the southern devil scorpion, native to his home state of Georgia. He assures me the name sounds more menacing than the sting feels.

"It's like a bee sting but less severe. I picked one up the wrong way when I was a kid and got stung on the finger. Then in college I was on one of my nature expeditions, laying in the dirt taking pictures of two scorpions. I didn't know a third was on the ground, so I rested my forearm on top of it and got stung. It wasn't squashed…" he hurried to reassure me, "it scurried off after! It was my fault in both cases."

Sam was always interested in wildlife; and as he delved deeper into his Muslim faith, his passion for animals grew.

"In Islam," he explained, "every single form of life on the planet, from a blade of grass to a human to a scorpion—every single thing—is purposely brought about on this earth. As humans with that in mind, we need to be less arrogant in how we are living and take care of these things that are necessary for us to exist."

In case you doubted that scorpions help humans to exist, the venom of one species is an ingredient in compound BLZ-100, which is undergoing tests as a kind of paint to guide surgeons to brain tumors for safe and complete removal.[14] In this way, scorpions save human lives.

There is a specific chapter in the Qur'an that inspired Sam, called "Surah An-Naml" ("The Ants") during which an ant warned her colony of an approaching army to prevent them from being crushed. Prophet Solomon, the leader of the army, smiled and rerouted the army around the ants, proving that he could communicate with and protect the smallest of animals.

"A lot of people don't think twice about squishing an ant, but this prophet behaved differently, and it had an impact on him." And on Sam.

There is also a hadith from Imam Ali, from Nahjul Balagha sermon 24, suggesting, in Sam's words, that "all the riches in the universe aren't worth oppressing even an ant." Or a scorpion.

I pondered my own dog-loving and birdwatching childhood and asked one final question as he pulled into the hospital parking lot.

"Do you have any pets, Sam?"

"Well, I almost bought a deathstalker scorpion once. I used to have a lot more venomous pets. Now I have a Socotra Island baboon tarantula. It's unknown how venomous they are——enough to make you feel miserable with horrible body aches but probably not lethal."

Sadly, Pickles, his six-eyed sand spider, passed away two years ago.

✳ ✳ ✳

Deathstalkers and tarantulas are both arachnids, arthropods with eight legs and a body divided into two segments. Pickles was an arachnid too, and if she looked anything like the pictures of sand spiders I found online, she not only had four pairs of long, jointed legs that spread across the ground like a handwoven net but also a body covered in tan velvet.

Now, I will admit, arachnids are the one group of beyond-human beings that *sometimes* give me a little shiver of fright upon seeing them. I am reminded of my time as an intern at a captive lemur facility in central Florida. Every few days I walked the outer perimeter of the fence to ensure that there were no downed branches on the electric wires or holes through which lemurs might escape. I never found anything wrong with the fence, but I was always met with an obstacle course of banana orb-weaver spiderwebs the size of umbrella canopies. Their artists were always perched in the center of the tapestry, at eye level, daring me to pass. I am constantly trying to unlearn this fear and fascinated by the fact that it often feels involuntary.

As I wonder whether I could have learned to bristle at the sight of a spider, I also remember the time when one of my parents tried to squish a spider in the living room of my childhood home. Upon impact, hundreds of babies exploded from the mother and spilled in ripples across our blue carpet. I had a similar experience years later in rural Indonesia after a friend removed a large spider from my bedroom wall with a broom. Just after I nestled in for the night and tucked the mosquito netting around my mattress, I discovered tiny clones of the mama spider on the floor, on the ceiling, and in every corner of the room. Now, there is a spider living under my desk as I type this who is quite welcome there. Another writing buddy. I'm working on it. "Lucas the Spider" of YouTube fame helps. So does pondering what it might feel like to *be* an arachnid.

At first, it is intimidating to wonder about how a critter like a scorpion perceives the world around them. For starters, they have multiple pairs of eyes in different locations on their head. To a human (and especially an anthropologist), a single pair of eyes is central to our sensory experience. The presence or absence of eye contact means so much to our species. We look into the eyes of our loved ones to connect. We avert our gaze so as not to threaten or stress another primate. Even when I look at a picture of another animal, I notice that my entry point into who they are is through their eyes. They are the portals, from our end of the experience anyway, to beyond-human connection. When we see two eyes looking back at our own, we see something familiar, some of ourselves in another being.

At first, I am stumped about how to connect with a scorpion because I don't know where to look. I struggle to interpret a scorpion's image when it appears that its eyes have been haphazardly sprinkled upon its front half by some clumsy arachnid creator with an overzealous saltshaker. There are eyes on the front of its face and on the top of its head. The longer I look, the less I am sure where the head even begins or ends! Then, I learn that despite the extra eyeballs, scorpions have relatively poor eyesight and instead rely on other senses. Their pectines, special appendages on their undersides, behind their legs, sense the world through chemical signals. These little limbs look like combs and function like antennae in other invertebrates, helping the scorpions to taste, feel, and smell their environment.[15] I might begin to embody the scorpion by removing my eyeglasses and shifting my focus to other senses.

✳ ✳ ✳

Vrschikasana is an inverted backbend. It is a forearm stand during which the back arches and hollows and the knees bend so the feet can reach toward the top of the head. The pose can stretch the front of the body, tone the spine, and strengthen the arms.[16] It is one of the poses, in my opinion, that most obviously mimics the animal after which it is named. My forearms along the ground resemble pedipalps, my legs a tail, and my feet the venom bulb. My toes do the occasional stinging.

I daresay renowned yogi B.K.S. Iyengar would have disagreed with me about pulling focus from the scorpion's sting. To him, this asana is a metaphor for striking negativity from our minds. He wrote,

> The head which is the seat of knowledge and power is also the seat of pride, anger, hatred, jealousy, intolerance, and malice. These emotions are more deadly than the poison which the scorpion carries in its sting. The yogi, by stamping on his head with his feet, attempts to eradicate these self-destroying emotions and passions. By kicking his head, he seeks to develop humility, calmness and tolerance and thus to be free of ego.[17]

Either way, I am doubtful that my feet will ever graze (much less stamp) my head in a handstand, resembling a striking scorpion. Not in this lifetime. No matter how many vrschikasana tutorials I watch, how many dolphin poses (a forearm version of downward-facing dog), forearm planks, or headless handstands I practice, I cannot touch my head with my feet while balancing upside-down on my arms. I am okay with this. Still, I work on my forearm stand at the wall, lifting my feet off the ground and tapping the solid support behind me for a few seconds at a time.

As my eyes look toward my hands in those quick bursts of scorpion, I can feel pectines between my elbows, recalculating gravity, recalibrating how I know to be animal in the world in barely perceptible increments of physical progress. A fraction of an inch of an arching spine. A nanosecond longer in an arm balance. A pause in acknowledgment and gratitude for the wolf spider scuttling out from underneath my prickly pear cactus as I weed my tiny yard. A tad more courage to live among arachnids in my own home, or to escort them outside with a drinking glass, a piece of paper, and some good, old-fashioned compassion. This is the antivenom. It is how, with the assistance of scorpions I may never meet alive or in person, I will counteract the toxins humans can inflict on their own kind and others. The venom from within telling me that to be "better" at yoga I should be able to touch my toes to my noggin while standing on my hands. The venom from without suggesting that I regulate my own emotions and facial expressions so that others feel comfortable even if I do not.

As much as becoming other animals through asana can help us to think about how they might perceive the world, we are always limited by being a particular kind of animal ourselves, and thus having limited perceptions of what other beings sense. It's not a lack, but an acknowledgment that we are one of them. We will never know exactly what it's like to be scorpion and neither will the scorpion know what it's like to be human.

Indeed, the greatest challenge is emotional, not physical. To truly embody this impressive creature in mind and in spirit, we must consider the rest of the scorpion's life: the behaviors other than striking and stinging that make them who they are. Consider their earnest search for tasty and nutritious meals, their lounging in cozy burrows, their occasional juddering and jitterbugging with potential mates, then caring for the still-soft bodies of their darling scorplings until they can care for themselves. We can imagine scorpions in other, more relaxing shapes, with their tails draped along the rocky ground or curled to the side as they rest, perched on a log. In slumbering scorpion pose.

My (in)ability to sting does not define me, just as the ability of the scorpion to sting does not define it. Yes, I am pensive, a little anxious, and a lot passionate, but I too can flirt and dance and sleep cozily curled; I can use my own pedipalps to grab a tasty bite of paneer and rice. Behind my sometimes serious and unsmiling exterior, there are pectines on my *mesosoma*, my vulnerable arachnid belly. Always grounded, close to the earth, they sense too much and feel too deeply. Sometimes, with my tail outstretched and relaxed behind me . . . that is all I can do.

Practice
MINDFUL NATURE WALKING

Go for a mindful nature walk, or what Victoria Loorz calls contemplative wandering.[18] Think of it as "being while walking" instead of "going for a walk." A meandering meditation. Wander outside with mindful attention, engaged with the landscape. Move at a speed that is slower than you normally travel. Hike a trail you know well, a short loop, or an out-and-back trail so it is impossible to get lost. You won't get too far.

Thich Nhat Hanh wrote about walking meditation:

> Suppose we are walking to a sacred place. We would walk quietly and take each gentle step with reverence. I propose that we walk this way every time we walk on the earth. The earth is sacred and we touch her with each step. . . . When we walk mindfully, we see the beauty and the wonder of the earth around us. . . . When we take mindful steps on the earth, our body and mind unite, and we unite with the earth. . . . Whenever we breathe, whenever we step, we are returning to the earth. . . . With each step we fully arrive in the present moment. Walk as if you are kissing the Earth with your feet.[19]

Bring nothing with you. No notebook, no camera, no phone (if you carry it for safety, switch it to "do not disturb" mode), no field guide. No destination. Walk in silence, slowly, with a smile. Go barefoot if it is safe to do so. Feel your feet as they touch the ground. Notice how gravity connects you to the earth with each step. Replace plans and expectations with pectines. Stop often, and take time to explore. Let your senses follow what interests them. Feel the grooves in the tree bark. Crunch a dead leaf in your fist and listen to the lively sound it makes. Smell the dirt. Squat down low. If something is bothering you (unpleasant smells or temperatures, itching, etc.), acknowledge how you feel, and remember that the sensation is impermanent. Be present with those sensations.

Peek under rocks. Notice the little critters like salamanders, spiders, centipedes, and roly-polys (pill bugs). Wonder about their lives, their experiences, their personalities, how many eyeballs they might have. Replace the rocks carefully, leaving them as you found them. Touch the lush patch of moss next to the rock and imagine the microscopic critters with otherworldly names: tardigrades, nematodes, and rotifers. How would you think differently about an arachnid if it was the first time you'd ever seen one?

Greet the tick (another arachnid!) crawling up your pant leg, all the while acknowledging and appreciating the fear you might feel in such close proximity to an animal we are taught to avoid for good reason. Try to connect to the tick with a *beginner's mind,* the Zen Buddhist concept of regarding the familiar with a combination of curiosity and lack of judgment. Witness this beyond-human being. A fellow animal on a quest for food. Then politely escort the tick off your body to eat elsewhere. You are forever connected to each other by this brief encounter, but sometimes our fears keep us safe.

Walk slowly on. With each step, try to focus on your experience in *this* moment and *this* place. Feel gratitude toward yourself for taking a walk in nature for your own well-being and that of the others around you. Happy trails, fellow animals!

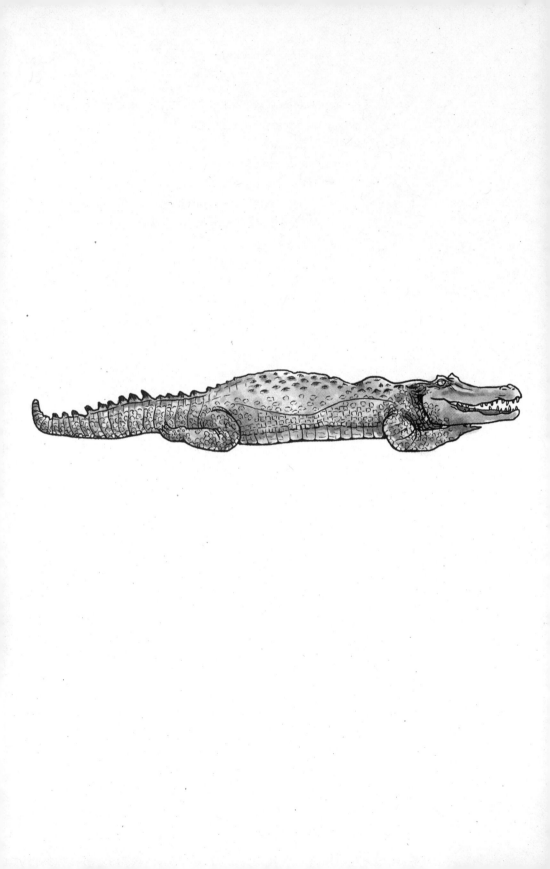

Chapter 9

NAKRA—CROCODILE

"Boo-ah-YAH," said the robot voice on the language learning app.

Then, in English, "Crocodile."

I was studying Malay to prepare for a summer abroad program in Borneo, the island habitat of three different species of crocodile, and the farthest yet I'd ever traveled from home. The first words I learned, and some of the only ones I still remember, were animal names.

A few months later, on a boat ride to Bako National Park on the coast of the South China Sea, I passed multiple signs from the Sarawak Forestry Corporation that read: *"AWAS* DANGER *Berhati-hati ada buaya.* Beware of crocodiles." *Awas* means "slow," but we drove past the sign so fast the letters blurred and we could barely read it. A few days later at Semenggoh Nature Reserve, a captive buaya, likely a saltwater crocodile, lay camouflaged against the dirty, concrete floor of her enclosure. I could see how, with her checkerboard pattern of brown splotches and black hexagons, she would easily disappear if she slunk into the murky water behind her. Her underside was pale, her front feet curiously small and dainty. The crocodile smile was real, although I couldn't decide if she had much to smile about. While she looked well fed, her enclosure seemed a far cry from the islands, coasts, tidal rivers, and freshwater marshes her free-ranging counterparts inhabited.[1] Perhaps she was being rehabilitated, later to be released back into the wild like the caiman, a cousin of the croc I met briefly, years later, in Ecuador.

My journal entry from that visit to Amazonia is a mess of bullet points, hearts, and scribbled exclamations. I felt at home in this humid jungle where the heavy rains stopped as suddenly as they started. Where the joyful over-whelm of numerous wildlife sightings was punctuated by warm and sticky midday naps. After dinner one night we departed for a tour of the lagoon with our guide, Eduardo.

"I have a surprise for you!" he said, carefully lowering a canvas bag into the floor of the canoe.

When we arrived, we witnessed the release of a confiscated white caiman, a species also called the spectacled caiman because of its promi-nent eye crests. Crocodiles and caimans share a branch of the reptile family tree with gharials—the narrow-nosed weirdos of the bunch—and alli-gators. Together, these four types of beyond-human beings make up the noble group of earth's crocodilians. They all share a similar scaly body type with long tails and snouts, an almost exclusively carnivorous diet,[2] and a semiaquatic lifestyle on the edges of bodies of water from small creeks to vast oceans.

We watched with headlamps as the caiman emerged from the sack and plunked to the bottom of the shallow water near the dock. There she rested, taking in her new surroundings under a beautiful full moon to a cacophony of frogs and insects, who replaced the day's earlier symphony of macaws, kingfishers, and hoatzins. Since caiman populations recovered from wide-spread slaughter for the skin trade, hunting of this common species is allowed throughout much of its range, where habitat loss is now the biggest threat to its survival. They might also be collected alive and sold into the pet trade because caimans are relatively small and easy to keep in captivity, compared to other crocodilians.[3] (I say "relatively" because no wild reptiles make good pets!) Despite a potentially stressful capture, confiscation, and journey confined in cage and canvas, this lucky caiman once again shared a habitat with anacondas, river dolphins, piranhas, and harpy eagles. Now, in a tributary of the Rio Napo, she was home.

❊ ❊ ❊

I come from the land of the alligator, north of the land of the crocodile.

In third grade, my class of Lewis Elementary Florida Panthers took a field trip to Silver Springs, the park of glass-bottom boat fame near Ocala.

"What do you remember about that trip," I asked my mom, who chaperoned, "other than the capybara earring debacle?"

I recalled standing with her, looking down at the largest rodents in the world, when her earring fell off and down into the enclosure. We waited patiently as a keeper helped us retrieve it. I remember my mom was more concerned about the animals' well-being than getting her jewelry back.

"Well, the park was in decent shape. It was very shady and had an 'old Florida' feel to it. Huge live oaks with lots of Spanish moss hanging from them."

I never thought much about Spanish moss until some out-of-state friends from college visited Tampa. I was so used to seeing it draped over limbs like tinsel on my grandparents' Christmas tree that when they asked, "What's that curly gray stuff?" it took me a minute to figure out what they were talking about.

The concept of old Florida feels a lot like the distinction between inland and coastal parts of the state. It is alligators and orange groves, not beaches and bikinis. A home, not a tourist destination. I realize that the Silver River is the perfect example of old Florida when I return to visit its source at Silver Springs as an adult. It is a magical place where the water is named for its crystal clarity through which you can see everything down to forty feet below, where water gushes from Mammoth Spring. During one glass-bottom boat tour, I saw turtles and mullet swimming above eel grass that flowed with the current like long locks of hair. Swamp ferns, like verdant feathers, tickled the water. A pair of wood ducks paddled toward the bank where cypress knees, knobbly and persistent, stood watch. Alligators, who varied in length from a few to about seven or eight feet, lounged on logs. One male gator visibly puffed up, trying to appear larger as the boat approached his basking spot on the bank. This social behavior is referred to as an inflated posture and serves as a visual signal to other alligators (and boats full of tourists) to demonstrate territoriality.[4]

The boat captain informed us that adult American alligators can grow up to fifteen feet long and that males are larger than females. Apparently, there is a handy trick for estimating gator length: each inch of the length from snout tip to eyes is approximately one foot of the gator's total length. This is especially useful when the head is the only part of the animal not submerged. Alligators are apex predators of the wetlands, swamps, marshes, ponds, and rivers in which they dwell, eating fish, birds, turtles, small mammals, and anything else they can catch and swallow whole.[5]

"Gators are an opportunity-type feeder," the boat captain explained.

"Oh, just like me!" said a tourist.

The boat captain shared a story from years ago. On a private tour a man was trying to take a picture of a twelve-foot gator, but he fell on top of him and got both of his legs bitten off. He survived the attack but sued the boat captain.

"But in court he didn't have a leg to stand on!" he concluded.

It seemed wrong to laugh about someone's misfortune, even if the story was exaggerated, but it's true that many injuries occur because people offer food or otherwise get too close—knowingly or not—to alligators. Responsible Floridians learn never to feed alligators and to be especially careful around bodies of water at dusk or after dark when gators hunt. We learn, sometimes the hard way, to keep pets and small children away from the water's edge. We may also learn not to zigzag if chased, as the myth suggests. Gators can sprint at nine miles per hour but have limited stamina. You are more likely to outrun them if you do so in a straight line. Just run fast![6]

"If you're swimming in freshwater in Florida, you're swimming with gators!" said the captain.

Indeed, people can be bitten or attacked simply for sharing the water with alligators and trying to enjoy a swim. I grew up with a respect for, but not a strong fear of, gators. My attitude seemed to perfectly mimic a biologist's description of one community's relationship with crocs in the Philippines. We share "elements of fear and reverence for [crocodilians] and a general attitude allowing humans and [crocodilians] to coexist."[7] Ancient Egyptians also held a dual perception of crocodiles "as a great natural power of which to be thankful as well as wary."[8] The countless gators I'd passed in motorboats or on kayaks over the years either disappeared underwater before either of us got too close or remained statue-still on the bank. It was mildly unsettling sometimes, but I always felt safe. Except for the time that I didn't.

On another trip to the Silver River, I was kayaking the Fort King Paddle Trail, a narrow canal dug out in the 1930s so a man named Colonel Tooey could take tourists on jungle cruise boat rides. I was paddling alone and searching the tree canopies for monkeys (that's a story for another book) when two young men floated into view.

"There's a big gator right there on your left," one said with a twang.

Big was an understatement. I had no choice but to float past him. We were so close to each other that I could have blown a dragonfly off his tail with a puff of my breath. Although I doubt he compared to the state's record length of over fourteen feet,[9] I can tell you the distance between his snout and his eyes: *too many inches!* Right after the gargantuan gator I saw a turtle the size of a coaster. This wily river sure loved to play with contrasts.

Then I got nervous. My choices were to return the way I came, passing that giant-ass gator again, or to paddle hard upstream at the headspring fighting against a current created by 5,800 gallons of gushing power per second (more doable than it sounds, but more effort than I had planned for). I looked back at his basking spot slowly, as I imagine people do when they are chased by zombies in the horror movies I don't watch. As it turns out, there was no time to decide what to do. He was no longer on the bank but swimming straight toward me down the middle of the narrow waterway. He passed me a mere three feet away and gave me the side-eye as he did so. I trembled with 90 percent fear and 10 percent awe.

Soon afterward, as I recovered from the close encounter, I saw the two men again.

"Freein' your mind alright?" one asked.

"I'm not usually scared of gators . . . but I was scared of that one!"

A few years later, Google alerted me to a news story reporting that a twelve-foot-long male alligator at the headwaters of the Silver River swam directly up to a woman on a stand-up paddleboard, and she used her paddle to push him away as he hissed at her.[10] As I continued to read the article, I realized there was a good chance that was the same gator I paddled past a few years prior. Multiple males, called bulls, of that size so close to the headspring are rare due to their territorial nature. In both cases a large gator demonstrated a lack of fear of humans—a behavior that is reinforced when feeding occurs. There is also a good chance this same gator was young and small when I visited as a child, almost thirty years ago. I felt sick watching the video embedded in the article because I knew what was coming next. Soon after the incident with the paddleboarder, the gator was shot in the head by a trapper contracted by the state. Unfortunately, because others likely fed him the way they feed monkeys and other park wildlife, he was killed. Alligators who learn to associate food with people are more likely to later approach and potentially attack them.[11] This is an all-too-common ending to a common story.

While to their prey and to the occasional quivering kayaker, alligators may be something to fear, they also function as valuable keystone species. Gators are ecosystem engineers who change the landscape to benefit hundreds of other species of plants and animals.[12] They burrow into the mud and create trails, providing freshwater habitat in dry areas; and in wet areas, their nest-building behaviors create a dry habitat for nesting birds and turtles.[13]

As I write this chapter, an alligator tooth sits on my nature altar next to an acorn and a beaver-chewed wood chip. It is the one remaining from a pair of earrings, a gift from an old friend who purchased them one morning after we brunched at Savvy Jack's restaurant. (Who doesn't need French toast and alligator tooth earrings from the same fine establishment?) The tooth is slightly curved with a tip as pointy as a recently sharpened pencil and a groove that would have helped the gator hang onto a still-thrashing almost-meal. Instead of chewing, crocodilians swallow their meals in whole chunks.[14] The tooth was clearly designed for gripping and crushing prey,[15] not for dangling from my earlobe.

I press the tooth into my skin with enough pressure to leave a small red dent at the tip of my finger, remembering that teeth were one of the ways I was trained to teach Busch Gardens guests the difference between crocodiles and alligators when I worked there as a zoo educator. Crocodiles show both their top and bottom sets of teeth when their mouths are closed, while on alligators, you can only see their top teeth. Alligators are also darker in color while crocodiles have more webbing on their feet. The only place you need to know any of this "in the wild" is in southern Florida, where the two species overlap.

The biggest difference of all, between gators and crocs, is habitat. While alligators are found in only two regions of the world, crocodiles are more widespread and diverse. At least thirteen species of crocodiles live across the globe throughout the Americas, Africa, and Australia, and on islands such as Madagascar and Papua New Guinea. Many crocodilians are named after their homes: American alligator, Nile crocodile, Cuban crocodile, saltwater crocodile, and the critically endangered Philippine crocodile. They live in freshwater, brackish water, and even thrive in saltwater habitats thanks to a salt excretion gland in their mouth.[16] A less scientific, more subjective difference I notice is that alligators have friendlier eyes than crocodiles, whose peepers appear more menacing. Perhaps those born in the land of the crocodile disagree.

Speaking of habitat, I had a recurring childhood dream about a river that was wide with dark greenish-brown water. I leaped from stump to stump across the endless ominous swamp, equally scared of the snarling pack of wild pigs that chased me and of falling into the water and drowning. Somewhere in between the clarity of the Silver River and the dreadful dark swamp of my nightmare is my home. I grew up less than half a mile from the fifty-four-mile-long Hillsborough River in a suburb of Tampa called Temple Terrace. As much as I love kayaking and looking down at manatees in spring-fed water, I also appreciate the blissful ignorance of not knowing what crocodilian lurks beneath my humble vessel. I came of age along the Hillsborough, where the water runs brown due to tannic acid released by decomposing plant matter, as it meandered—never far away.

※ ※ ※

Nakrasana, crocodile pose, does not do justice to crocodilian anatomy. They "are large, low, and long reptiles that live in aquatic environments," wrote Zach Fitzner,[17] and they have been this way for a couple hundred million years.[18] With their sensitive snouts, thick skin, and armor-like osteoderms that help regulate their body temperature,[19] crocodilians are an evolutionary marvel. Their muscular bodies never stop growing, and their choppers replace themselves tooth after tooth, well into adulthood. Crocodiles have a notch on their upper snout in which their longest bottom tooth snugly fits.[20]

In contrast, nakrasana is not physically complicated. It is my default urge of existence to lie prone like a crocodilian basking on a sunny log or floating in a marsh assuming a "minimum exposure posture."[21] They are perfectly built for it. In the pose, my legs externally rotate, the inner arches of my feet rest on the floor, and my forehead is supported by pillowed fists. My shoulders are tented. It is, uniquely, a gentle backbend that allows you to face the earth and turn inward. Practiced in moderation, the effect of the pose can be intuitive and restful.[22] Eventually, though, my crocodile tendencies send me to the chiropractor.

"How do you sleep?" the practitioner asks at the beginning of my first appointment.

"On my stomach."

He winces and squeezes his eyes shut and shakes his head. It's all very dramatic. Apparently, now that I'm in my thirties, if I like my neck, back, and shoulders to function without causing me pain, I shouldn't sleep on my belly.

* * *

I am fascinated by families who stay in one place for multiple generations. My great-grandmother, then my grandparents, then my parents left their home states, and I did too. My children will not be born where I was. It makes me wonder to what extent our ideas of home are cultural, passed down and learned from our loved ones. I was not—and am not—always a proud Floridian. I grew up hating the beach because of the sand and the heat and instead lusted after Colorado's Rocky Mountains. I think my hesitance to love Florida used to be due to the fear that I would get stuck there, living forever among the giant palmetto bugs and 1-800-ASK-GARY billboards. (Those personal injury lawyers are a different kind of predator.) I just always knew I was bound to move on. As I write this, I am living in the fourth state I've lived in since I left Florida. My brother also had to leave the state and return, to better understand it.

"In Florida, with the geography and topography, you're in it and it's hard to be an observer. Unlike out west with vistas and timberline and elevation changes. But the sheer amount of subtropical biodiversity here is overwhelming," he said.

It's hard to see what you're in the middle of. Crocodilians spend their entire lives bellies to the ground or peering out from under the water's surface. They are also unable to see the changes in topography that we observe from above or from the outside or after being away from home for some time (except when they climb trees, a behavior crocodiles and alligators have both engaged in on occasion).[23] They sense their prey, each other, and the landscape in other ways. In addition to vision, hearing, and smell that benefit crocodilians both in and out of the water, they all have sensory nerve bundles called ISOs spread throughout their bodies to help them navigate in the most unclear aquatic conditions.[24] Crocodilians can also sense the earth's magnetic field, making relocation efforts (for example, from a golf course or a retention pond to a more remote habitat) challenging and often unsuccessful. Researchers have resorted to transporting the animals with a magnet attached to their heads in an attempt to disrupt this ability.[25] Animals know where home is.

In some ways, I feel like a visitor in my home state these days. (On a recent trip, I went to the drugstore to buy aloe vera gel for my sunburn ... like a damn tourist!) I start to suspect I feel that way because I appreciate Florida again. If landscapes collect memories,[26] I return like a treasure hunter to admire the way squirrels scurry in spirals down oaks dressed in Spanish moss. I reminisce about buying hot boiled peanuts in a Styrofoam cup at a roadside stand. Weirdly enough, I even miss those couple of weeks every year when fuzzy, alien caterpillars descended upon our backyard. And oh, how I enjoy the diversity of avian life! On a recent visit I counted more than ten species of birds between two sips of coffee on my parents' patio.

So, if Floridians, wherever they happen to live, don't stick up for Florida, then who will? Since I left, I defend my hometown and the entire state from everyone else I meet. Florida is that relative only other family members can talk badly about—if an outsider does, then I get defensive. In many ways, Tampa does still feel like home: When the plane touches down at TIA, it feels welcoming like no other airport does. I am a vegetarian who regularly craves a Cuban sandwich (and occasionally caves). I paid vague attention the last time the Lightning played for the Stanley Cup, despite not being a hockey fan; and I always know when it's Gasparilla, Tampa's annual, pirate-themed version of Mardi Gras, and feel a little festive from afar.

I've wrangled with the concept of *home* for so long that I've often felt envious of nomadic people whose idea of home is less tied to a single physical place. Back in northern Virginia where I now live, after watching the Netflix series *Tiger King*, I lay facedown on the floor with my head on my hands. My dog Meeko lay next to my yoga mat licking his stuffed alligator toy. It's complicated being from Florida. The rest of the country both vacations there and relentlessly mocks the state for looking like a gun and a penis, and for eccentric characters such as Carole Baskin and Florida Man, the stereotypical news character archetype who highlights the quirky characters who call the state home.

The Marjorie, a nonprofit news organization reporting on environmental and social justice issues in the state, rebelled against this trend by leading a "Reclaim Florida Woman" campaign in honor of three influential Florida ladies named Marjorie (Kinnan Rawlings, Harris Carr, and Stoneman Douglas).[27] If caring about the well-being of others and the environment is what it's all about, then consider me a proud Florida Woman. Whenever the culture of my home state does not resonate, the nature and wildlife do. You can't beat anhingas and panthers, roseate spoonbills, and multiple species of crocodilians. I may live elsewhere now, but I constantly impose characteristics of Florida onto my current home. There is always the possibility of a gator in the human-made lakes and ponds of the mid-Atlantic piedmont. There is always the call of a limpkin just beyond the traffic noise from I-66.

I asked my husband how he thinks I feel about Florida, and he said, "You hate it!"

I asked my best friend the same question and she said, "You love it!"

This is the contradiction of being from Florida.

Yoga helps. Most simply, nakrasana is me embodying an animal that shares my love of landscapes warm, humid, wet, and sometimes a little salty. When I practice it, the bullshit disappears like bottled water from the grocery store shelves during yet another hurricane forecast. In crocodile pose, I am still. A minimum exposure posture, indeed. I am a cold-blooded ectotherm, preferring a solid 85 degrees Fahrenheit ambient temperature. I am camouflaged and no one can bother me, but I am not unaware of my surroundings. My body senses my environment in new ways and I expertly navigate murky waters and cloudy conceptions of where I'm from. With my head down, I feel the perfectly complicated combination of the clear waters of the Silver River and the murky swamp of my childhood dreamscape. The comfort of home mixed with the shame of leaving it behind. As fellow Florida Woman Eila Carrico writes in *The Other Side of the River*, "My feet continue to carry me away from Florida, but they cannot seem to escape the swamp."[28] For alligators, crocodiles, and me, Florida is home. And whenever I am unsure, there is nakrasana.

Practice
FINDING HOME IN THE BODY

Go lie down in your bed or the most comfortable place you can find. Get cozy under the covers. Hang out on your back, moving or resting, then roll onto your belly. Inhabit your body and notice what emotions arise. Maybe your body is telling you to put on a certain song and sing. Maybe your home is a person. Let them know. Let the concept of home be as simple or complex as you are prepared to sense right now. Ponder the following questions:

Where is home for you, and why?

What is the temperature of your home, the smell of the air, the ambient sounds?

What does the scenery look like out the window?

What movements make you nostalgic?

What yoga pose or movement feels like home in your body?

What animal best represents your home, and how do they move?

To inspire nostalgia, look at old family photographs, type your childhood address into Google Earth, search for a local list of native wildlife. May you feel at home in your body no matter how far from your geographic home you find yourself.

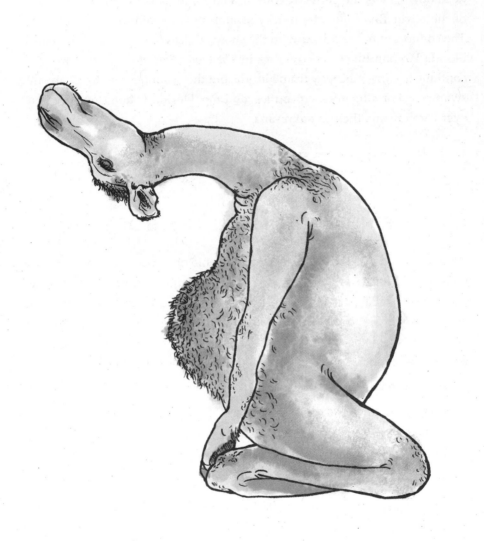

Chapter 10

USTRA—CAMEL

We kneel to protest or to pray, to plead or to propose marriage. We kneel to begin to become camel. It sounds simple, but the action can carry a lot of emotional weight, while the physical weight of the body is concentrated mostly on delicate knees. For ustrasana, I make my place of kneeling soft like desert sand by using a blanket underneath me for cushioning.

My hips hover directly above my knees, and the tops of my feet press into the floor. I lift my chest toward the sky and let my heart open and expand, working my shoulders down behind me. This subtle movement, again, is deceptively simple. Opening the heart is intense and vulnerable. It can break us open, revealing a stash of strength and beauty inside that we may have forgotten existed. In fact, according to some sources, the word *camel* comes from the Arabic *jamil*, meaning "beauty."[1] Becoming camel can't happen without this opening.

Watching videos of camels lying down, I am dubious how this tall and strangely proportioned creature will ever transition from standing to lying with any grace. The legs are too long, and the weight too wonkily distributed. There is a pause before the action, which is then initiated from the camel's head and neck as in ustrasana. Her front and back feet are so centrally positioned under her body that they are almost touching. The camel lowers her head toward the ground, seeming to redistribute weight in preparation for the folding of her legs. Then, her front knees bend, and the camel kneels with feet underneath her and the weight of her hump thrown forward. For a split second it looks more like falling and I fear for the camel's bones and joints, but her front half stills. After the briefest pause for subtle shifting, her back legs fold like an accordion and the camel cow settles.

There is a terrifying moment for me, right before a backbend, when I doubt I can do it at all. Kneeling and upright, I am certain I cannot reach back and touch my heels, but I am always wrong. The body's tools support me: my bones, my muscles, my breath. After reaching my spine long, I place my palms behind my hips. I can start to feel the backbend happening even before I initiate the arching movement. As I open through my chest and shoulders, anchoring my hands to my hips is the bridge to remembering how to backbend.

When I arch my back, my hips sneak forward, and I return them to their position directly above my knees, focusing on the movement of my torso curving toward the wall behind me. Yoga helps us remember that we have animal bodies as we arch backward to mimic the camel in a movement that can benefit the mobility of the spine and help release upper back tension, not to mention stretch the front of the body.[2]

I slide my hands toward the ground and clasp my heels. My arms, like long, spindly camel legs, are what support the weight of my torso. The biggest challenge of all is managing the heavy, bulbous thing that is my head. Camels would have this problem too if it weren't for their long, muscular necks. To protect mine, I stay in control and prevent the weight of my head from dropping behind me.

Finally, I am here. Breathing, opening, deepening in a backbend. The front of my body expands while my lower back stays roomy and uncrunched. No straw can harm this camel's back! Depending on whom you ask, ustrasana resembles a camel standing, in the process of lying down, or just its hump. I imagine that I am a wild camel grazing on succulent grasses and browsing thorny shrubs.[3] I am leggy yet sure-footed and my silhouette shows perfect curves that mimic the patterns of the windblown sand upon which I stand. I release my heels and unfold to return to kneeling, back to where I began. After un-cameling in body, I feel energized and invigorated.

❉ ❉ ❉

Not only yoga, but also handcrafting with animal fibers, can connect us in unique ways to the beyond-human beings from which our materials come. We never create alone. From the tools we use to the lives that inspire our creation, nature can be a part of our crafting lives. In Barbara Kingsolver's brilliant essay about knitting, the sweater starts with the sheep.[4] What I create begins with a camel.

Wild Bactrian camels have two humps, tall legs, shaggy coats, long faces, and strange-looking feet. Today, most are domesticated, but a few wild flocks survive in small numbers in China and Mongolia.[5] They are critically endangered, and little is known about their behavior. Unlike the more common single-humped dromedary camels, they live in colder climates and experience some of the most extreme temperature changes and harshest weather conditions of any mammal.[6] In winter, the wild camels travel vast distances, eating snow when water is unavailable. During this time, domesticated Bactrian camels produce fiber that people collect and spin into yarn.

Camels have two types of hair: a guard layer on top and an undercoat called camel down, which is used as wool. Bactrian camel hair is softer and warmer than sheep wool,[7] and it is so well insulating that Berbers make tents and clothing from it.[8] The camels molt naturally, so they don't have to be shorn as sheep do. I woolgather about wool gathering, imagining an afternoon in the Gobi Desert, collecting camel down among spindly legs that keep bodies elevated above hot sand and cold snow.[9] I find tufts of soft fiber nestled in among hardy shrubs and bunches of grass baking in the sun.

There is a certain pride in knowing where—and whom—your yarn comes from. Alpacas are in the camelid family along with llamas, guanacos, and vicuñas. I decide to visit some at the Butterfly Hill Farm Store in Waterford, Virginia. There, alpaca owners Gerry and Catie Dutcher sell locally raised products and artisan crafts.

I meet seven Huacaya alpacas on an overcast day. They range in color from off-white to dark brown and wear long tufts of hair that rain down from the edges of their ears. Their breath warms my hands as they take pellets from my palm with incisors like shovels. One of the alpacas, finally satiated, lies down at the edge of the fence and I touch her soft fleece. My entire pointer finger sinks down to the knuckle.

Inside the shop, I munch on homemade peanut brittle and cherry cookies as the conversation turns to camels.

"I spun some baby camel wool once," Catie says, "I thought, 'Oh this'll be so much fun!'" She shakes her head and whispers, "I hated it!"

We both laugh. Spinning is the process of turning raw wool into a string-like form that can then be knit, crocheted, or woven into products. The fibers of wool are literally spun together as if by magic, by hand or with a spinning wheel or machine, pulled from a clump of wool.

"The fibers are really short!" she explains. "You need a different piece of equipment to spin camel wool."

"When you spin, do you think about the animals?" I ask.

"I do, especially when I spin specific animals. You think about when they were a baby, or when they had a baby. It's almost like having children. I knit a shawl with Willow's wool, and then she passed away, so I never decided to sell the shawl. As I'm working on it, I'm thinking about her, so to get rid of it is to get rid of that last memory of her."

I can hear the loss in Catie's voice.

"It's kind of the end of an era when you lose your founding animals. She was the first one [whose wool] I ever spun. I spun her for my aunt because her husband had just died. When my aunt died, I got the scarf back that she knit from that yarn. It's so comforting to me when I wear it now. In that respect, there's a connection both to my family history and to my animal history."

Inevitably, there is heartache and loss involved when we share our lives with animals, but creating something with the wool they produce leaves tangible and enduring comforts that honor their memory.

I purchase a couple skeins of yarn and thank the alpacas who grew it on my way out. While leaving, my car gets stuck in the mud and Gerry tows me out with his truck, smiling. I wave goodbye as my mud-covered tires hit the asphalt of Charles Town Pike.

After this visit I am inspired, so I sign into Etsy to order a skein of 100 percent hand-spun camel yarn and eagerly await its delivery. When it arrives, I tear open the package, stuff my face into the fuzzy bundle, and inhale deeply. The smell of natural yarn is one of life's greatest pleasures. I stroke the soft fibers that resemble the color of milky chai. Apparently camel fiber feels like merino and acts like cashmere,[10] but I don't have these frames of reference. I only know the feeling of it between my fingers.

People refer to a collection of unknit yarn as a stash and that is where my ball of camel wool waits as I ponder what to make with it. Initially, I want to crochet a little camel in the Japanese *amigurumi* style, which is characterized by small, stuffed crocheted or knit dolls, but I change my mind as the yarn sits idle on my craft desk. I decide instead to make something that I will use in a manner similar to how the camel used her own wool. A simple cowl knitting project will encourage mindfulness and result in something that will warm me as I wear it close to my skin.

Depending on how yarn is "put up," or packaged, it may not be immediately ready to use. To make my yarn knittable I need to first unwind it from its original form (a loosely looped and then twisted form, or hank) and wind it into a ball so that it unravels again easily as I work. It is a simple yet integral part of the process. Knitting shops will wind your yarn for you, but I prefer to do it myself. Unwinding by hand allows me to touch every inch of the fiber, to get to know the yarn in this form before turning it into something else. I imagine the oils from my fingers mixing with the lanolin-like substance that covers camel wool to keep their coats dry and free from harmful bacteria. I place the circle of yarn around my knees, sitting so it is taut enough to stay in place while I wind and watch the Winter Olympics. A figure skater performs a trick called a camel spin as I unravel and wind, unravel and wind, opening my heart to the beauty of the yarn and its potential to become something beautiful in a different form.

Imperfections are abundant in handspun yarn, I notice as I wind; but instead of bothering me, the stray strands, varying thickness, knots, and fuzzy bits connect me to the spinner. Knitting and other crafts not only connect us to fiber-producing animals, but also to artisans from around the world and throughout history who have worked with similar tools and techniques. The spinner may be the first person to add imperfection to the piece, but she is not the last. Opening up to allow ourselves to make mistakes—in life, yoga, spinning, or knitting—is so valuable. The mistakes are not something to undo or to hide. They are visible reminders that we aren't perfect. They become a part of the piece and part of us. Still beings of beauty. Jamil.

I fear beginning a knitting project as I do initiating a backbend. I've been admiring the yarn, now wound with care into an imperfect sphere, for weeks. Touching it, smelling it, but not knitting it. Then I remind myself that working with the yarn, not looking at it, better honors the animal who provided the fiber. So, it is time to cast on, the process of putting the yarn onto the needles in the proper sequence of useful tangles. It forms the edge of the piece with a foundation of loops into which I will knit. I find the tail end and panic as predicted.

Holding my tools sparks my memory. I use Takumi single-pointed bamboo knitting needles, size 8mm. When they click together it makes a gentle, hollow sound like the thud of two-toed camel feet leaving lily-pad-shaped tracks in damp sand. Just as the yarn is more important than the knitting itself, the associated tools are as precious as your favorite spatula or your comfiest pair of shoes.

Yes, okay, I *can* knit. I form a slipknot and begin to cast on, holding a strand of camel in my right hand. With a few delicate flicks of my wrist, I cast on one stitch. Then two. I soon lose count. Now I remember. When I cast on, I cast a spell. Instead of herbs and incantations I hold sticks and string, infused with nature, to anchor me before I begin to create human clothing from camel "clothing." I don't knit with a pattern. My projects are guided, stich-to-stitch, by curiosity and intuition that blows in like a storm through the Mongolian steppe.

Sometimes we stash away yarn, sometimes memories. In high school, a classmate taught me how to knit at a cafe one afternoon. We weren't close friends. It was the only time we hung out, just the two of us, but knitting brings people together like that. I bought chunky, rainbow-colored yarn and thick needles for my first lesson. The finished product was a gaudy, triangle-shaped scarf, but I was thrilled.

When I lived in San Diego during graduate school, a friend taught me how to crochet. A group of anthropology students gathered every Wednesday evening at a coffee shop for yarn night. Hooks in hand we made hats, granny square potholders, and coffee cup cozies while we talked about course assignments and fieldwork travel plans. Yarn, and the evenings spent in the company of friends as we all worked it through our hands, was my "sturdy lifeboat."[11]

I can't recall the impulse that made me want to learn to knit in the first place. No one in my family can remember any relatives who knit, although my ancestors lived in mountainous, wool-producing places and surely needed warm clothes to wear. Like relearning to cast on and remembering how to backbend, I had to relearn how to knit after generations of forgetting. Now, I make clothing out of string like silk-spinning spiders and nest-weaving orioles. I use sticks as tools like chimpanzees and crows do while foraging for food. I arch backward, open my heart, and make the shape of a camel with my body, bending one vertebra at a time. I knit one stitch, one row, one ancestral memory, at a time.

I believe that, to some extent, we have all experienced another kind of collective forgetting: We forget that we are animal. In many camel-keeping cultures, the animals are known for their impressive memories, and their cognitive abilities are often compared to human children or dogs. They remember those who treat them well and mourn them when they are gone.[12] A story from Morocco, about a camel who reportedly killed a teenage boy who beat it,[13] demonstrates how they remember those who mistreat them too.

Around camelids it helps to be calm and compassionate, but it's beneficial while knitting too. Instead of attention to the breath, it is attention to each stitch. One after the other. It is a repetitive, life-giving practice that can keep us mindful. If you want it to. Knitting can also be mindless. I could spend the rest of my life knitting rectangular things, letting my hands move while my mind rests, and be as happy as a freshly shed camel in summer. It's all about balance. Sometimes I am so tense with needles in hand that my shoulders can be found hiding behind my earlobes. I worry about the size of the piece, whether I've missed a stitch, or if I've purchased enough yarn. Knitting *can* be relaxing, but it's not always.

Camel pose is not relaxing in the moment either. Sometimes there is a time lag between our practice and the beneficial effects of it. I cannot feel the improvements to my blood circulation or kidney function as my fingertips brush my heels. Nor can I see new muscle definition in my legs or glutes as soon as I unbend. "Trust Allah but tether your camel," says an Islamic proverb paraphrased from a hadith.[14] In knitting and in ustrasana we work with our bodies and minds together to find that feeling that everything is smoothly working together, seeking that balance between effort, flow, and trust in the process.

Finally, it is time to cast off, to remove my finished piece from the needles. I sew the ends together at the seam with little yarn to spare. With my cowl complete, I wear it right away. I feel accomplished and connected. When we craft with animal fibers, we work with beyond-human beings to create something that neither of us could create alone. Now I have a cozy camel cowl to protect my neck, keeping it safe and warm as I open my throat in ustrasana. I connected my breath to the stitches and pondered the personality of the camel whose wool wove between my fingers. Every cowl I make and every ustrasana I practice is a blend of human and camel.

※ ※ ※

Camels are often referred to as "ships of the desert" because of their capacity to transport people and goods across arid landscapes, across oceans of sand. Both types of camels are famously adapted for living in harsh desert climates. In addition to having humps, they barely sweat and their eyelids and nostrils close during heavy winds. They can eat thorny plants and drink large amounts of water quickly at one time after detecting the microbes with their keen sense of smell. Oval-shaped blood cells help them recover from extreme dehydration, and they even, to some extent, drink the moisture from their breath thanks to specialized nostril grooves.[15]

Camels were domesticated around 4000 BCE,[16] and humans have lived alongside them for thousands of years. To many, camels are also an anchor to cultural tradition and to a kind of livelihood in which human and animal are woven together with the tightest of stitches. In fact, I could not find much information about camels that was not directly linked to their uses for humans. Camel expert Bernard Faye wrote, "No other domestic animal is able to provide such a variety of uses for human populations."[17] Camels have been and still are sources of food, medicine, shelter, fiber and clothing, transportation, luck and blessings, fuel, art, labor, fertilizer, and entertainment.[18] Their milk provides potential health benefits for people with autism, diabetes, lactose intolerance, and more.[19] In some parts of the world, camels even function as libraries, bringing books to children in rural areas of Kenya and Mongolia.[20]

The one-humped dromedary camel features prominently in lore and legend. I hate the phrase "beast of burden," but it came up again and again in my research. In *How the Camel Got His Hump* by Rudyard Kipling, the camel was too lazy to work for humans, so he voiced his rebellion in the form of a single, grumpy "Humph!" So that's what he got. I must say, good for him for refusing to work only for the benefit of people; and good for the friendly *djinn*, or spirit, who used his magic for quite a useful punishment, as camel humps store fat and allow them a better chance of surviving in their native habitats.[21] According to an Indian tale, camels originally had five legs but struggled to walk, so the god Shiva took the extra leg and turned it into a hump instead.[22] The Raika people of Rajasthan who share this story believe they were created by Shiva to care for camels, and the animals are still integral to their culture and livelihood.[23]

I am guilty of this viewing of the camel through a human-use lens too. My experience with camels through a product, only a small part of the whole animal, is representative of the available literature about them. While many farmers, ranchers, and scientists like Temple Grandin have pondered the lives and well-being of individual cows, I find no such accounts of personal and meaningful relationships with humans and camels. This doesn't mean that they don't exist, but suggests that few have been written in or translated into English. Little scientific research has been conducted as well.[24] There are papers galore on the camel meat and milk industry, but resources on the behavior and ecology of wild or domestic camels are few. It turns out, there are limits to the extent to which we can connect with camels if we only ever engage with a part of them.

Furthermore, due to the "environmentally friendly" nature of camel farming and the animals' ability to survive in areas that experience severe drought, the practice is touted as an increasingly relevant solution for climate change adaptation.[25] Because of the camel's many uses alive and in the form of food, others promote the potential of camel farming to address food insecurity and economic depression in rural and remote locations.[26] Few of these reports include consideration of the camels as individual beings, except the work of a group of veterinarians in Rajasthan working to ensure that camels have access to medical treatment, anesthesia for painful procedures, comfortable harnesses and related equipment, and reflectors to prevent collisions with vehicles.[27]

I fly through Abu Dhabi every time I visit India, and if the souvenirs in the airport are any indication, it is the camel capital of the world. That, combined with the view of endless camel habitat out of the airplane window during takeoff and landing, makes me yearn to leave the duty-free dates in the literal dust and go meet a camel for myself. Finally, one day I got that chance. Not in Abu Dhabi, but in rural northern Virginia. When I arrived at the farm and saw the dromedary in his paddock from afar, I noticed three large sand-colored humps. Two were piles of hay and Aladdin's single hump formed the third.

I approached and greeted him with a small handful of hay "cookies" that he took with a wobbly bottom lip and chewed with conviction. The whole process culminated in a swallow that I could see and hear in a series of gulping grunts. He wore a faded red halter that his owner, Jen Cossette, clipped a leather leash to before we watched him stand up. His long face ended in a snout as satisfying to touch as a horse's. A tiny cloud of dust poofed from his hair when I stroked him on the neck as Jen explained that his coat gets thicker in the fall and is sheared in the early spring, although he sheds some naturally too. I found a clump of camel hair on the ground that was coarse and flecked with bits of hay.

"You can keep it!" Jen laughed.

I put it in the back seat of my car, and while giving a friend a ride home from dinner soon after my visit I had to say, "Don't sit on my tuft of camel hair!"

Aladdin was about fifteen years old, fourteen hundred pounds, and seven feet tall at the hump when I met him. He was born in 2007, making him barely middle-aged in camel years. Jen got him when he was one month old and bottle-fed him with the help of her young son, who would play hide-and-seek with Aladdin, disappearing behind barrels in the paddock until he was discovered.

"I actually meant to get a zebra, but I came back with Aladdin," Jen says, smiling. "He doesn't really know he's a camel; I think he's a little bit different because of the way I've spoiled him. He's more like a dog, really!"

Taking Aladdin on a walk was not much of a walk. He ambled into the shade of a big tree nearby and started munching on greenery, using his lips like fingers to pull down and manipulate branches and pluck individual leaves.

"Are you a giraffe?" Jen asked him.

Goats bleated and multiple farm dogs ran around the camel's legs as he browsed unperturbed. In between bites he sniffed everything at nose level and regarded his surroundings with large, kind eyes protected by a curtain of enviable lashes.

"Aladdin, you're so curious!" I said to him, and he reacted to hearing his name by looking over at me and down at my hand, no doubt hopeful for another hay cookie. He found only my notebook, which he decided to taste instead.

Aladdin is clearly attached to Jen. At one point, she handed me the end of the leash and entered the barn to get more treats. He watched her leave and waited patiently for her to return, keeping an eye on the door into which she disappeared.

As amiable as Aladdin is, he is not only Jen's companion. He is an integral part of the business she started twenty years ago called Pony To Go. The camel is one of a motley menagerie that also includes bunnies, ducks, chickens, alpacas, ponies, sheep, a skink, a bearded dragon, a hedgehog, goats, and a few snakes. These animals make up a traveling petting zoo that may visit casinos, nativity scenes, weddings, festivals, children's birthday parties, and more. For most of his life, Aladdin has also spent the winter holiday season at Mount Vernon, the historic home of George Washington outside of Washington DC, where he greets visitors and represents the camel that the first U.S. president paid to have visit his estate in December of 1787.[28]

"What's the one thing everyone wants to know when they meet Aladdin?" I wonder.

"Everybody asks me if he spits. He doesn't spit . . . except when the vet comes!" Jen shares that she plans to retire soon and sell Aladdin to a trusted longtime client.

"I love doing this and sharing him with people, but it's not easy work and I'm getting older. I'm gonna miss him so much . . . he's like my family. I know I'm gonna cry my eyes out when he leaves."

"Well, he obviously loves you!" I offer. I have no doubt that when Aladdin moves on to different pastures that he will miss Jen as much as she will miss him, but how do you comfort someone who has to say goodbye to their beloved camel?

Before leaving, I got to watch Jen spray Aladdin with the hose after we returned him to his paddock. His joy was obvious as he moved so the spout of water would hit specific places on his back and hump. It wasn't long before he began the laborious process of lying down and I watched from the other side of the fence as his back legs trembled and buckled. Once he was down there, the play was effortless. Aladdin thrashed and rolled on his side in the camel-sized mud puddle, like a dog "scent rolling" in deer poop with glee. Then he flipped to the other side to do it all over again, smearing mud equally and evenly on both sides of his body, which pressed against the fence as he rolled, straining the wooden slats with his enthusiasm.

My favorite picture Jen took of Aladdin and me shows me holding his leash and looking up at his face while he looks over my head and past me into the distance at something else. Did I fail at connecting with a camel? I only knitted with a small piece of a whole Bactrian camel being. And according to many sources, ustrasana indeed represents only part of the whole animal. Although ustrasana may mimic just the hump and we may knit with only their wool, my camelid musings and meetings have reminded me that to unify we cannot deny the initial separateness. This is the first terrifying step, like starting a backbend or a knitting project when you've forgotten how to get the yarn onto your needles or doubted that you can open your heart. Acknowledging the separate parts, unwinding before rewinding, and arching the back inch by intentional inch, eventually results in becoming camel. Or wearing camel, as the hairs at the base of my neck mingle with strands of another being. Crafting with the fibers of other animals has its limitations, but it's quite an intimate act. We wear part of an animal against our own skin. Although it is only part of them, through the process of making and wearing, they become a part of *us* in a unique way.

Camels are useful to humans, yes, but that's not why they smile. According to a Muslim proverb, camels are the only beings that know the hundredth name of God. One of the other ninety-nine names that fits the camel well is al-Hadi, the guide. Camels help guide us in yoga and in creative projects, always walking alongside us, or carrying us and our yoga props and knitting needles, "to the goal of unity with Unity."[29] Allah and that tethered camel . . . those two are in cahoots.

Practice
NATURE JOURNALING

You don't have to be a knitter to connect with nature in a creative or crafty way. Nature journaling is another useful tool for exploring the natural world. It is accessible for anyone who has a piece of paper and a pencil on hand. Although the idea can feel overwhelming at first, the practice is meant to be a fun and creative way to focus your attention and inspire curiosity as you make observations in nature. In *The Laws Guide to Nature Drawing and Journaling,* John Muir Laws writes:

> I feel understanding, care, and compassion when I journal and turn deep attention to nature. Love of the natural world is the spring that waters commitment to stewardship: protecting and being responsible for something— in this case, wildness and biodiversity everywhere. As journaling pulls you deep into connection with the world, this connection may lead you to action. Look for ways to make a difference where you live. Find and join a community of stewards or be the catalyst for work to start on a cause you feel strongly about. Nature will restore you as you restore nature.[30]

I have been nature journaling for a few years, and the style of my pages depends a lot on my mood. Sometimes a page will be covered in words, sometimes in pictures, sometimes a chaotic combination of both. Sometimes I use color and sometimes I don't. The materials I have on hand include a collection of old colored pencils, a regular No. 2 pencil, a kneaded eraser, a white vinyl eraser, two archival-quality fine-line markers, and a cheap journal with blank pages.

DO:

- Start with plants or other immobile objects (rocks, landscapes, fungi, etc.). They are less likely to walk, fly, or slither away as you observe them.

- Use John Muir Laws's three main prompts to begin, or whenever you feel stuck:

  - What do you notice?

  - What do you wonder?

  - What does it remind you of?

- Use words and pictures to complement and enhance each other.

- Follow the work of fellow nature journalers on social media for motivation and inspiration.

DON'T

- Let your fears about not being "artistic enough" hinder your progress. It doesn't matter what your completed pages look like as long as you connected more deeply with the source of your inspiration and learned something new in the process.

- Compare the pages in your journal to other people's pages. Your journal should not look like anyone else's—it should look like yours!

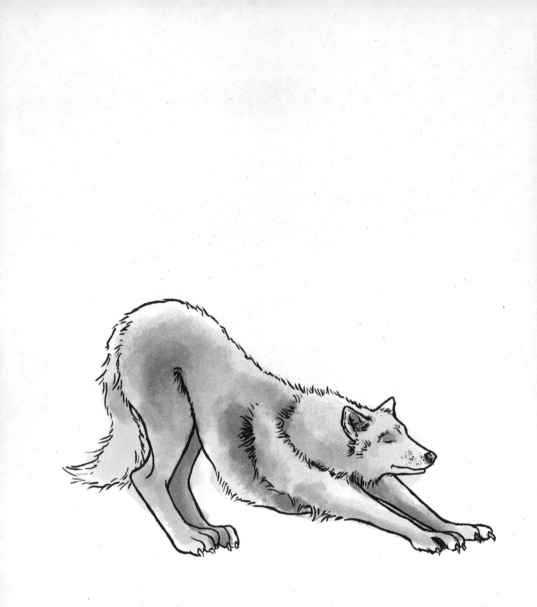

Chapter 11

SVANA—DOG

Don't worry. The (domestic) dog doesn't die in this chapter. I am not willing to accept that "my" dog, Meeko, will ever die. But many coyotes and wolves—also dogs—will, and did, and still do. Humans love certain dogs and despise others to a degree that howls hypocrisy. Relationships with our canine companions are often affectionate, yet they change dramatically when the dogs live on the edges of human existence instead of pampered inside our homes.

Ethologists Wolfgang Schleidt and Michael Shalter claimed that wolves domesticated us as much as we domesticated wolves,[1] during a process that began between ten and forty thousand years ago.[2] Whether or not this theory holds up in our ever-changing understanding of the topic, the idea of a reciprocal process, a mutual coevolution, resonates with me. Our ancestors were part of a multispecies becoming into what our relationship with canines is today, for better or worse. Pondering the object of the leash, only briefly, demonstrates how "domination, domestication, and love are deeply entangled" in the words of anthropologist Anna Tsing.[3]

We know of one famous wolf from his tangled encounter with St. Francis and the people of Gubbio, a small town in the Apennine Mountains of Italy. As the story goes, a wolf was causing problems for the town's residents, feeding on livestock, and sometimes attacking people. One night St. Francis traveled to the edge of the forest to confront the wolf, who immediately approached with teeth bared and hackles raised. When St. Francis held up his hand, the wolf froze and lay down at his feet. St. Francis could see that the wolf was hungry and just as scared as the townspeople. He arranged for the townspeople to feed the animal while the wolf wagged its tail in agreement not to attack any humans or livestock again. The people and wolf grew fond of each other and when the wolf died, the town mourned a collective loss.[4]

In this story, the wolf reacted differently toward St. Francis because St. Francis reacted differently toward the wolf. The two beings were curious about, and experienced unexpected behavior from, each other. They desired to understand each other and had the capacity for empathy and compassion. In fact, the wolf's described behavior was consistent with that of other carnivores who are more likely to prey upon livestock and attack humans—those who are injured, old, or otherwise struggling to hunt. Furthermore, wolves are social animals who cooperate with and help each other, coordinate hunting efforts, and feed and care for young other than their own, so they are required to read the faces and body language of other animals to navigate pack social dynamics.[5] We observe this in domestic dogs too, in the ways they pay such close attention to the movements of others. For example, some dogs develop a limp in response to a leg injury in a human to whom they are attuned. Even yawn contagion jumps species boundaries from humans to dogs.[6] "So why did that wolf lie down at Francis's feet?" Steve Kotler asks. "Because . . . unity is contagious, and why bother attacking yourself?"[7] The wolf was a canine yogi.

The wolf–human relationship is a curious phenomenon. Having worked in the field of human–wildlife conflict and coexistence for years, I know that no beyond-human being is more polarizing or more divisive than the wolf. While wolves have changed with their environment over millennia, it seems that humans are stuck in a time lag regarding how we think about and treat these wild canines so entangled in our lives, landscapes, histories, ecologies, and folklore. Interestingly, wolves evoke the worst in humans from both extreme ends of the coexistence spectrum: unproductive animal welfare fanaticism and misappropriation of the term *spirit animal* by non-Indigenous folks on one end, and indiscriminate predator extermination and scapegoating a single animal for the modern challenges of ranching on the other end. With wolf-dog ownership lurking awkwardly somewhere in between.

Our collective, historic hatred of predators led to the regional extinction of large, apex carnivores like wolves, cougars, and grizzly bears. Gray wolves, for example, once ranged across much of North America, but by the mid-1900s, they were found, in the U.S., only in small pockets along the Canadian border.[8] Subsequently, a phenomenon called *mesopredator release* occurred. Smaller, often omnivorous predators like raccoons, skunks, and foxes experienced increases in population size. Coyotes are another example of a mesopredator who began to thrive when wolves were nearly eradicated. A cynic might say people then transferred their hate to the next largest predator still around.

The book *Coyote America: A Natural and Supernatural History* by Dan Flores made me cry on an airplane. I don't even know where I was flying to or from, but I know that I was alone, sitting in a window seat and reading something I knew would break my heart. And it did, right there on the plane with my body twisted toward the dim sparkle of streetlamps far below. I hid my silent sobs from the stranger seated next to me as I read about coyotes and their status as the "most persecuted large mammal in American history," hated more than rattlesnakes, rats, and cockroaches, according to a survey conducted by Yale University in the 1980s. They were treated as such.[9]

The late 1800s would have been the worst time to be a coyote in North America. Inhumane trapping, shooting, and poisons called *predacides* were used, resulting in indiscriminate and excruciating wildlife suffering. The killing was not limited to North America; it was a tragic, global phenomenon. Dholes, also known as Asiatic wild dogs, in southern India are similar to North American canids in social structure and behavior. Like coyotes they were "slaughtered mercilessly" by colonizers invading the land and wishing to hunt. They were shot, poisoned, vilified, and referred to as "bloody killers."[10]

In my nonprofit work helping landowners manage problems like tree-felling and flooding caused by beavers, the coyote is another animal that I consider to be a human-coexistence–challenged "sister species" to the North American beaver. The disturbing attempts to exterminate coyotes, motivated by strong, internalized emotion, feel crueler to me than the largely economically motivated near-eradication of beavers. While millions of beavers died so people could wear waterproof top hats, coyote hatred was visceral and deliberate. Beaver pelts were currency, but coyotes were the enemy. Aside from economics, another influence may be the difference in human perceptions of predator versus prey species. Regardless, coyotes and beavers both survived and recovered from nothing less than a concerted effort to erase each species from our landscapes.

Coyotes are many complicated things to the people who coexist with them. Even within the Navajo tradition, coyotes represent varying roles from heroes and healers to tricksters and thieves. While there is a distinction between Coyote the deity and coyote the animal, they share similar characteristics like boldness, inquisitiveness, stubbornness, and power.[11] Richard Louv, the journalist best known for writing about the concept of *nature deficit disorder*, calls animals like coyotes "betweens."[12] They live in the city and the country and everywhere in between, especially on the edges of definable habitat types. Living along cultural *and* ecological boundaries as they do, coyotes occupy the spaces in between our definitions of urban and rural, and forest and farmland, crossing highways and existing alongside millions of people mostly undetected. They are also genetically in between wolf and dog as their genome contains the DNA of both.

Today, coyotes are somewhat less persecuted than in the past, but no less resilient. They thrive in our midst despite the many changes humans make to the landscape, adding new survival challenges such as roads and subdivisions. People fear coyotes because of their reputation, deserved or not, for attacking livestock (especially sheep and goats)[13] in rural areas and people and pets in more developed habitats. In one article from 2004, the authors refer to coyote attacks as "an increasing suburban problem" and list all reported coyote attacks on humans in California from 1978 to 2003. About one-third of the eighty-nine attacks targeted children younger than eighteen years of age.[14] While pets make up very little of a coyote's total diet, the proportions do vary by location. For example, Seattle coyotes seem to enjoy cat meat more than those who live in Chicago.[15] Coyotes are more likely to feed on pets due to human behaviors such as failing to secure trash, feeding pets outside, and not cleaning up fallen birdseed and fruit.[16] They might also attack pets because they feel threatened by the presence of another mesopredator with whom they might be competing for food.

When coyotes are hunted and trapped in response to these concerns, they react by producing larger litters and reproducing earlier in life. These are the same solutions coyotes used to employ when other apex predators applied the pressure. The adaptation they used to survive wolf predation is the same one they use to thrive today despite efforts to control coyote populations. So, not only is the "solution" to the coyote "problem" cruel—it is utterly ineffective. "All along," wrote Flores, "coyotes had been saving themselves."[17]

Years ago, I observed one coyote in the middle of a suburban San Diego street late at night, and another at the edge of a marsh on Christmas morning in Florida, both animals no more than a stone's throw from multiple occupied homes. Then, while writing this chapter, I visited Rocky Mountain National Park on a day trip while vacationing in Colorado. My husband and I observed moose in the lush montane habitat of the park's lower elevations and watched marmots chirping atop lichen-smeared rocks, above the treeline in the alpine tundra. A pika perched like a statue, relying on its exquisite camouflage and rock-like build. A bull elk grazed, unfazed, mere feet from a traffic jam accumulating in his antlered honor. It was an incredible day of wildlife watching. In our final moments within the park's boundary, we drove back toward Grand Lake through an area that had recently burned. The tree trunks were charred, black sticks, many fallen and askew. The hillsides were scorched gray. The only animal I saw, trotting through the grass—the only vegetation that had already returned—was a coyote. She loped away from the road, and if it wasn't for the movement, I never would have spotted her. When I brought my binoculars to my eyes, I saw the coyote's ears first. She turned to look at me for a second and disappeared into a burnt world.

✳ ✳ ✳

While the human–canine relationship is complicated, all I have for wild, domestic, and everything-in-between dogs is love. It is as simple and clichéd as that. It's not exactly riveting stuff—a person who loves dogs, especially "their own." You can buy the phrase "dog lover" plastered across almost anything, and the hashtag #doglover has 87 million posts on Instagram at the time of this writing. I don't have the slightest idea how to write about "my" dog in any meaningful way, because many have tried before me, and because love is all there is. But . . .

I awoke on the morning of Wednesday, January 27, 2010, assuming it would be another normal day of college classes. At some point in the afternoon, I got a voicemail from my mom inviting me over for dinner that night. When I arrived, my aunt and uncle were there too. I noticed them acting strange from the beginning, but then my dad poured a glass of my favorite white wine and said, "Cheers!"

"What are we toasting?"

No one answered.

"You guys are acting weird!" I said.

My aunt's head swiveled as she grinned at me and then looked into the living room. Finally, I followed her gaze and saw this little puppy timidly walking toward us.

"Oh my God! Who is that?"

Everyone was laughing as the realization hit me: I finally had a puppy! One unexpected sip of wine later and I was a "dog mom." He was six weeks old. A little black-and-white, thick-striped half Shih Tzu, half Yorkie-Poo with a blond muzzle, blond front paws, and a severe yet charming underbite. He was the cutest creature I had ever seen. I kept thinking, *Oh my gosh, I have a puppy!* It was surreal.

I have loved Meeko ever since that night. Since that moment when I looked over and saw his tiny body on the living room floor and it dawned on me that I was allowed to love this creature with all of my being, because no one else would ever love him more. I love the way he smells on bath day, of Fritos and maple syrup. I love scratching him in just the right spot so he straightens his hind leg while I yell, *"Turkey leg!"* I love walking outside with him, following as he pursues scent trails, his nose leading the way. I love the way he agrees to snuggle only when I put my smartphone down, encouraging me to be present with him, and then, the way the curve of his body fits perfectly in the "cuddle cove" of my own, his head against my heart. I love to watch his paws twitch in synchrony with soft yelps as he dreams. Curled up on the carpet behind me as I type these words, Meeko is a "good dog." And yet, neither the word *good* nor the word *dog* comes close to describing the extraordinary being he is.

Good dog. What a redundant phrase, an embarrassing understatement. Being "good" is a dog's default form of existence. It is our own as well, yet we blunder through life striving to feel something that remotely resembles canine-caliber "good." It is challenging to recall and embrace our default goodness when we are full of fears both evolutionary and new. Even the harshest, most violent opinions of wild dogs, what Dan Flores calls an "instinctive carnivore loathing,"[18] can be explained by our genetic memories as prey instead of predator, experiences of fear like that exhibited by the people of Gubbio before St. Francis came along. When we say "good dog" to our canine companions, we are really reassuring ourselves that we are capable of such goodness and love. We are. And this is what makes the human-loves-a-dog story remarkable after all. I am only capable of such goodness because of Meeko. Dogs call us into love.

Meeko has been the most consistent companion in my life for the last thirteen years. The longest we were ever apart was when I spent nine months conducting research for my master's degree in Indonesia, where an undercurrent of my entire experience was not getting too attached to animals. I call this modulated attachment *care-switching*, drawing from the linguistic concept of *code-switching*, the practice of changing the way one speaks based on context.[19] Instead, we change the degree to which we care for the well-being of animals depending on the situation in which we find ourselves. It is this same emotional survival skill that allows me to work with beavers that might be trapped and killed. I keep an intentionally curated emotional distance from individual beavers so I can continue the work that will ultimately prevent the same fate for future beavers.

One day during fieldwork in Indonesia, while checking camera traps near a watermelon garden, my research partner and I found a young puppy near our motorbike. I fed him a peanut butter snack bar, and we drove away. After checking another camera, we were surprised to find him near the tires of the motorbike again. He must have followed our scent trail snaking along the rocky ground and the sound of the bike's motor, both detectable to canine noses and ears. My heart ached a little as we drove away that second and final time. I knew there was nothing I could do for this puppy. Even if Ibu Haji, with whom I lived, allowed me to keep a dog in her house, there would be no one willing to care for him a few months later when I went home. At that point it would be worse for both of us.

As we sped away from the garden, I kept my eyes trained on the road ahead and fantasized about a dog shelter where strays were taken in, neutered or spayed, trained to act as guard dogs to prevent wildlife from raiding gardens, and adopted out to local farmers. It wouldn't help that dog, but it might help others, and people too! A primatology colleague faced a similar choice and eventually had to leave behind a dog she raised from puppyhood at the end of her research trip. Watching Naruto the dog watch her walk down the road with all her bags for the last time broke my heart—and likely, his. I don't blame her—we simply had different strategies for coping with the idea of animal suffering while in an unusual situation.

When I returned home, I was beside myself with excitement to see Meeko again. My parents brought him to the airport to pick me up. I was a little worried he would be mad at me at first, but when we saw each other at baggage claim we were as thrilled to meet in real life as we were in all my anticipatory daydreams of the reunion. Despite feeling overjoyed to see my dog and my family again, I had a severe case of reverse culture shock, and it took me a while to readjust, to feel like I belonged in my old life. Months later, cuddled in bed with Meeko, I thought of the puppy from the garden and started to sob. I was convinced that I left that dog to die. I realized that my animal-related emotions were calibrated back to life in the U.S. as I felt my heart breaking all those months later. I had finally, fully "come home."

We care-switch all the time with animals, especially when it comes to canines, experiencing what I call the "dognitive dissonance" demonstrated by people's inconsistent treatment of domestic dogs, coyotes, and wolves. The term *cognitive dissonance* was coined by a psychologist in 1957 to acknowledge discrepancies in "pairs of cognitions"[20]—in this case, the treatment of a beloved pet dog compared with negative attitudes and potential mistreatment of wild coyotes or wolves. The underlying discomfort arising from this contradiction, the "dognitive dissonance," leads the person to seek out only information that confirms their belief, for example, that coyotes are scary or dangerous. I care-switch with dogs, so I can't blame other people for it, but there are different levels of behavioral contradiction. Care-switching requires some level of cognitive dissonance to exist at all. We do this also with the animals we eat and wear versus those we point to in cutesy board books with young children as we "moo" and "cock-a-doodle-doo." Sharing a planet with dogs, we feel extremes of emotion from intense hatred and fear to deep sorrow when we lose them (even if they were not "ours" to lose) to unbridled joy when we love them.

❊ ❊ ❊

Years ago, as dusk fell, I stood at the base of a mountain in Colorado look-ing up at the motionless chairlift and silent ski slopes, empty except for a golden retriever and his human companion. The human threw a toy and the dog ran, leapt, and played with such pure, tangible joy that my eyes welled up with hot tears. I have never forgotten it. Maybe I recognized some semblance of the same pleasure I got from skiing down those same slopes a few hours before. I am often so anxious I could rub a worry stone out of existence, but with skis attached to my feet, fresh snow beneath them, and the Rocky Mountains surrounding me like old friends, I too am joyful. The mountains where I live now are smaller and slightly less skiable, but luckily, I have yoga to express that joy through my physical body. I play on my mat like a golden retriever with a tennis ball coated in slobber and sunset-hued snow crystals.

Kneeling in table pose, I walk my palms forward one hand's length. I curl my toes under and lift my hips. Downward-facing dog, *adho mukha sva-nasana*, is the "one-pose-cures-all asana," according to expert yoga teacher Judith Hanson Lasater.[21] My body forms a triangular shape, "like a dog stretching after a nap."[22] Above the hips I am happy. I wiggle them, wag-ging my tail. My spine reaches long, and I press up and out of my shoulders with the confidence of a retriever fetching her favorite stick. This inverted asana is meant to stretch the spine, strengthen the arms and hands, open the chest, improve circulation, and counter fatigue.[23] My head dangles, relaxed, and I shake it slowly from side to side the way Meeko keeps his gaze, his *drishti*, on a moving treat target.

Below the hips, I need to move. I pedal my feet, walking the dog, as they say. My heels reach toward the floor like a mutt on a harness and leash, straining ever-forward in pursuit of squirrelly scents; yet my knees remain bent. My hamstrings whine; my calves whimper. Downward-facing dog represents the stretch that dogs often take while standing up after resting, but the shape our bodies make in this pose also resembles a common canine social behavior called a play-bow. To soothe the tightness in the backs of my legs, I think "play-bow" and the whole pose changes. There are subtle adjustments to my posture and transformative effects on my affinity for the pose. My lips fetch an upside-down smile. I take myself less seriously, finding playfulness.

I remember back to the first yoga class I ever took, when the teacher told us that adho mukha svanasana was a "resting pose." *Huh?* I tried to pant through the pain in my shoulders and strain in my hamstrings. I recognize this suggestion now as one of the small ways in which a yoga teacher's language can serve to make the practice less accessible to people of different physical abilities or spiritual goals. While her intent may have been to motivate her students, this posture is not restful for a dog either. The stretch and the play-bow both occur in quick, few-second bouts followed by other equally adorable stretches or social behaviors, sometimes directly after a period of rest. Fifteen years into my asana practice, downward-facing dog still doesn't feel like a resting pose.

Wolves, coyotes, and domestic dogs all engage in the play-bow behavior, although frequency and function differ between species.[24] You may remember that, as the world was heading into the uncharted waters of the global coronavirus pandemic, a camera-trap video of a coyote and a badger went viral, giving us all a needed sense of camaraderie. The coyote play-bowed and wagged his tail before the badger followed him into a culvert and they trotted off together.[25] These two species are known to hunt together but, in addition to better predation success, this video was the first to suggest that they might also benefit socially from the enjoyment of each other's company.[26] Play doesn't immediately fill the belly, but it does enrich the lives of human and beyond-human beings.

Playfulness, to me, is "three-legged dog," during which, from adho mukha svanasana, I lift one leg behind me. The act of un-squaring my hips unlocks my hamstrings and my grounded heel drops to touch the earth with ease.

"Heel. Good dog."

But my lifted leg is flying. It is liberated. Off-leash. It bends and straightens, testing my three-legged foundation. Many dogs who have lost a limb to accident or illness are able to run and play and maintain a quality of life that matches those of their four-legged companions. A friend of mine is "owned by," in her words, a three-legged dog named Huckleberry Hank the Hop Along Hound. He was hit by a car before being adopted, and his right hind leg was amputated. With one less limb, he frolics and plays like any other dog, sometimes standing on his remaining hind leg when he gets excited about dinnertime.

The Yoga Sutras of Patanjali claim, "You call something a dog because it has a dog's body. The spirit in a dog and a human is the same."[27] If it is true that dog "owners" begin to look like their dogs, then it may also be true that if we practice adho mukha svanasana enough we will start to look in our bodies, feel in our minds, and be in our spirits more like dogs. To sense our goodness in unique ways. While practicing wild asana we change our perspective of poses we have been practicing, in some cases, for many years. In turn, the poses change us. Just as human-dog coevolution and domestication was a reciprocal process that changed everyone involved, through yoga we become more animal, more ourselves, more connected to other beings. We are a part of each other. Richard Louv wrote, "Through shared experiences and emotional bonding over time, humans and other animals, domestic and wild, come to see the world in similar ways. We change each other over time."[28] Our yoga practice can help us to embody the qualities of morality, intelligence, loyalty, playfulness, community-mindedness, and attunement to others that our canine companions on any part of the domesticated–wild spectrum do. We all play-bow. It doesn't matter what it looks like from the outside, in the physical sense. It matters what it feels like, and what essence of love, playfulness, and goodness we embody with our tails in the air and our heels wherever they hover.

Dog sanctuary owner Steve Kotler wrote, "The real reason I think dogs are sacred and dog rescue a path to enlightenment—because it's a path where play is not only encouraged but rewarded."[29] During kids' yoga, we howl in adho mukha svanasana. Adults, too, should give this a try. People howled every night at a certain time during the pandemic: to thank essential workers, as an emotional release, or to create a bit of playful music in community. The howl unifies. It is yoga. It is the sutra, the thread, of canine song that connects all dog beings and us. May we heed the advice of psychoanalyst C.P. Estés in *Women Who Run with the Wolves*, "Let us return now, wild . . . howling, laughing, singing up The One who loves us so."[30]

Good dog.

Practice

DOWNWARD-FACING DOGS

By using yoga asana to explore the boundaries within our own minds between domestic dogs, coyotes, and wolves, we can begin to question our deeply held biases and canine-related contradictions. Settle into your yoga space with a few mindful breaths. Have paper and something to write with available nearby.

1. Practice adho mukha svanasana by beginning on your hands and knees in table pose with hips over knees, shoulders over wrists, and a neutral spine. Move your hands one handprint forward. Curl your toes under and lift your hips. Bend your knees so you can extend your spine long as you relax your neck and let your head dangle. Engage the muscles in the backs of your legs by imagining your heels reaching toward the floor. Press into all your fingertips, keep the elbows softly bent, and push up and out of your shoulders. Stay in downward-facing dog pose, for as many breaths as is comfortable.

2. Move from adho mukha svanasana into child's pose by shifting your weight toward your hands and gently dropping your knees to the ground. Uncurl your toes and shift your hips back toward your heels. Guide your chest and forehead toward the floor, reaching your arms long in front of you.

3. Write in your journal about what it felt like to embody the dog.

4. Practice downward-facing coyote pose, for as many breaths as is comfortable. Refer to the instructions in step 1—nothing about the asana itself changes. Simply embody a coyote instead of a domestic dog.

5. Practice child's pose, referring to the instructions in step 2.

6. Write in your journal about what it felt like to embody the coyote.

7. Practice downward-facing wolf pose, for as many breaths as is comfortable. Still, nothing about the asana changes. Simply embody a wolf instead of a coyote.

8. Practice child's pose.

9. Write in your journal about what it felt like to embody the wolf.

10. Play-bow. There are no instructions. Listen to your body. Howl your heart out.

11. Ponder the following questions and continue to journal for as long as you are inspired:

    In what ways did the pose feel different each time you embodied a different kind of dog?

    In what ways did your relationship to the pose change from dog to coyote to wolf?

    What personal biases, if any, did these variations of *svanasana* evoke?

    In what ways does asana encourage you to think about any of these beings in different ways?

    Did you learn anything about yourself from practicing the same pose but changing your perspective about the beyond-human being it represents?

    What does it feel like to be in between dog and coyote? Coyote and wolf? Between wolf and human?

Consider that, during any given asana practice, depending on what you need in your life at that moment, you may embody the domestic dog, the coyote, or the wolf. All three are svana.

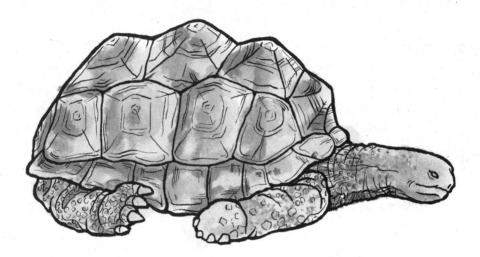

Chapter 12
KURMA—
TORTOISE/TURTLE

Imagine an animal so important, so influential, that they are literally the foundation of human life in multiple cultures from the Americas to Asia to Africa. Indigenous peoples in North America, such as the Iroquois Confederacy, revere turtles as totems or symbols for multiple clans. As Maurice Dennis told his friend Joseph Bruchac, "The turtle is the symbol of the entire earth. We walk upon the turtle's back."[1] The Zuni interact with their ancestors through ceremonies in which tortoises are reincarnations of the dead, the *otherselves*.[2] In *Braiding Sweetgrass*, Robin Wall Kimmerer retells the Indigenous story of Skywoman, who falls from above onto a turtle upon whose shell the earth is created.[3] I've seen turtle statues at temples in places as different as Dharamshala and Cincinnati. From Hinduism to Santería to Indigenous oral tradition, turtles are integral to earth's creation.

It's no wonder journalist Peter Laufer said, "Everyone has a turtle story."[4]

I say, why settle for one? I want to collect hundreds—no, thousands—of turtle stories, my own and others', eggs like dented ping-pong balls collected in an expertly excavated nest of sand. You can never have too many turtle stories. Here are a few.

❋ ❋ ❋

Jeffrey Popp, co-director of the Terrapin Institute, has worked with terrapins and other turtles for over twenty years. When I asked him for his turtle story he said, "Who doesn't love a turtle?"

"Why turtles, though?" I pressed, as part of my lifetime quest to get to the bottom of those "irrational species-specific devotions" science author Mary Roach wrote about in *Fuzz*.[5]

Jeff's turtle story began with a childhood love of reptiles and amphibians. He wasn't allowed to have a dog, but at age five he got his first pet—a Toad named Toady.

At first, his reaction was, "What am I gonna do with a toad? I want a dog!"

He eventually came around to the charm of the toad and they spent five years in each other's company. Then, after a routine pesticide treatment at the vacation house where they were staying in Deep Creek Lake, Toady tragically died.

"We had a little ceremony for him. After that I knew I wanted to be involved with wildlife. People love turtles, but they still think herps are unintelligent." (*Herps* is short for *herpetofauna*, a term that distinguishes reptiles and amphibians from other animals.)

After caring for Toady, Jeff knew differently. As a teenager, he participated in his state's head-starting program for diamondback terrapins, a gorgeous species whose skin is spotted and whose shells are covered in delicate swirls. Jeff cared for three hatchlings—Larry, Mo, and Curly—for an entire school year and kept them in an aquarium in his bedroom.

One day, Jeff's family came home from dinner to find Curly stuck, "literally between a rock and a hard place . . . underwater and wedged between a rock and the glass," he explained. "Terrapins don't understand glass, but they have to breathe air from the surface. We thought he was dead. He was totally limp!"

Jeff grabbed him from the water, lay down on his bed, and put Curly on his chest. He delivered gentle squeezes to expel water from the tiny terrapin. At one point, Curly lifted his head and put it back down.

Jeff thought, "Okay, well, maybe this is working!" So, he continued. Sure enough, after an hour or so, he managed to get the water out of Curly's lungs. He survived, and they eventually released all three terrapins back into the wild. After that personal connection, Jeff was hooked on terrapins.

"We still know so little about their behaviors," Jeff says in a voice full of fascination and respect.

Now, his favorite thing to do is to go to a mudflat or a nesting beach to watch a female diamondback terrapin in the process of laying her eggs.

At first, she hangs out in the water for a couple of hours to make sure it's safe as she scouts for predators and ensures that the coast is, quite literally, clear. Normally, she can slip away into the water if she needs to escape danger, but on dry land, she is especially vulnerable. She climbs out of the water and searches meticulously for the perfect place to lay her eggs. She knows to lay above high tide and at the base of plants, but specifically not near grasses that can puncture the eggshells. Then she digs. Once she starts laying, she doesn't stop until there are at least five, and sometimes more than twenty, eggs in the nest. Jeff shares that, in recent years, the Eastern shore has lost a lot of sandy beach nesting habitat, and sometimes the next best place is a gravel driveway that bloodies the female's feet as she digs.

"You can see it in her eyes. The sun is out, and it's blazing hot, but she's so dedicated to making sure the eggs survive, to creating that next generation. She uses her back feet to move the eggs off to one side to lay more, then she does a great job of covering them. If you speed up the footage it looks like a Riverdance."

She uses sand and grass to fill the hole and pats it down with her plastron, the bottom part of her shell. Then, she's off.

❊ ❊ ❊

"I am from as far away from the ocean as you can get, so seeing sea turtles felt like meeting a mythical creature!"

After receiving a bachelor's degree in environmental science and geographic information systems, twenty-four-year-old Nebraska native Rachael Green spent two months as a wildlife technician in Costa Rica on a sea turtle nesting project. She described herself as a white American girl "ready to save the turtles" when she arrived. She and a team of two other technicians would walk twelve-mile transects each night. The beach they patrolled, on a remote part of the island, was a nesting habitat for four species of sea turtle (leatherback, hawksbill, green, and loggerhead) who nested in overlapping phases throughout the season.

"It was amazing! I got really fit and tripped over a lot of coconuts," she laughs.

They couldn't use headlamps to navigate, as light may have adver-
tised nest locations to poachers who also patrolled the beaches in the dark.
When she started this work, Rachael had "terrible, horrible" ideas in her
head about poachers. After a couple of weeks on the job, her team was
approached by a man with a flashlight.

The poacher spoke to them in Spanish, "Hi, how are you?"

They chit-chatted, and then went their separate ways.

"He was so nice, and he looked like a dad. The realization felt like a bonk
on the head. This was just a person!"

She learned that, for some of the local people, the collection of sea turtles
and their eggs for food was part of the culture and had been for a long time.
She explained that just because sea turtles are now endangered due to a complex variation of global factors, that doesn't turn a fisherman into an enemy of
conservation. She also saw litter washing up on the beaches from elsewhere,
a factor as much or more to blame for declining sea turtle populations than
poaching. After learning from her mistakes, Rachael dove deep into social science. Her encounter with this fellow human, who was nothing like the stereo-
types she once held about poachers, changed her view of the animals too.

The hawksbills were the species actively nesting when Rachael was
there. As they walked the beach each evening, the team searched for tracks,
the turtles themselves, and the locations of nests. If a female was in the
process of nesting, the techs would try to get an accurate egg count as little
white globes were added to her pile.

One night, a female hawksbill had already laid her clutch of eggs and
was using her back flippers to cover the eggs when she was spotted by the
team. Sand was being flung into Rachael's face as she struggled with the mea-
suring tape, trying to record the carapace (the top part of the shell) dimensions. As she gently brushed the creature with her fingers, she disturbed
some bioluminescent algae in the wet sand, and the turtle glowed a beautiful fairy blue, leaving subtle streaks on the intricately mottled shell.

"I still think about that sometimes," Rachael shares in a soft, reveren-
tial tone.

Now, Rachael has a master's degree and has worked as a wildlife conservationist on projects with grassland birds, bats, and African wild dogs.

She is conscious of the harm caused by "parachute science," when Western researchers travel to other countries to conserve wildlife without a nuanced understanding of the local, cultural context. Instead, Rachael studies the human dimensions of human–wildlife coexistence and approaches conservation with culturally sensitive strategies and an open mind. Her turtle story was quite powerful in shaping the way she thinks about humans and other animals. It changed the course of her career and her life.

❉ ❉ ❉

Danna Hinderle has been a tortoise biologist in California for more than twenty years. At first, she wasn't drawn to the tortoises themselves, but to the fun and flexible lifestyle of hiking, camping, traveling, and working with awesome people. Now, she considers it a privilege to share space with the beyond-human "mellow vegetarians" who have taught her so much.

"Tortoises have shown me how to better engage with the world," she explains.

They have demonstrated, at different times, patience, independence, curiosity, gentleness, and stubbornness.

"And they sleep a lot, which I'm totally into!"

Her favorite turtle story is from her graduate fieldwork, during which she was radio-tracking four hundred critically endangered Mojave Desert tortoises within a twenty-square-mile area. She was walking a route about fifteen kilometers long—a big sweeping loop through granite rock formations like you might see in Joshua Tree National Park. She climbed over and under colossal, weathered boulders.

"How did the tortoise even get here?" she thought as she struggled to locate a route to get there herself.

One tortoise evaded the team for so long that he was logged as missing in the database. Everyone coveted the job of searching for the missing individual as it required perseverance, a sense of adventure, and the eventual satisfaction of uncovering the animal's location. Like hide-and-seek but way cooler (and hotter).

One 113-degree day in July, Danna was tracking the missing tortoise among the boulders. Previously, she used a particular cave for shelter during hot weather, and on this trip, she spent a few hours lunching and resting inside it.

"It had solid shade, a delightfully cool, sandy bottom, and no wind. It was truly the perfect nap spot."

As she was packing up her gear to leave, she heard something deep within the cave, "the distinct sound of a tortoise shell against rock." There she discovered the burrow of the missing tortoise tucked far back into the cave.

"It struck me that this tortoise was just going about its life—napping in the shade on a hot day like I was—completely oblivious to the dozens of hours my colleagues and I had spent looking for it. Not a care in the world."

❊ ❊ ❊

Jeannie Martin has worked as a sea turtle biologist and conservationist for the last eighteen years, also studying the effects of coastal and marine debris like cigarette butts and other single-use plastics on our oceans' wildlife. One individual that stands out in her memory is a juvenile green sea turtle, nicknamed "M," who was found on the Florida coast in the winter of 2013. She was discovered with fishing line wrapped around her front flipper and tethered to a picnic table. The fishing line caused multiple open wounds and infections that led to a weakened state known as cold-stunning, which occurs when the animal is exposed to low temperatures for an extended period of time.

"M was a mess . . . an adorable mess!" Jeannie recalled.

After surgery to amputate M's flipper, Jeannie was on the veterinary team who even helped the turtle breathe as she recovered, blowing air into a bag, through a tube, and into M's body at a rate of one breath every two minutes. Over time, M's condition improved, and she moved into a deeper tank so staff could monitor her progress to determine if, because of her missing flipper, she could be returned to the wild. Over the course of her stay at the rehabilitation center, she passed swimming and hunting tests, proving that one missing flipper wouldn't prevent her from living a full life.

"What was it like breathing for a turtle?" I couldn't resist asking.

"Exhausting." She paused, "You know, I never thought of it that way. When you're in the moment you don't think about it because you're so focused on the task at hand. It's always been more of a clinical thing than an emotional thing. Yes, the whole wildlife rehabilitation process is an emotional experience fueled by passion, but you also have to maintain a professional distance."

Not only is it heartbreaking if the patient can't be saved (and Jeannie spoke of some cases that "went south" and resulted in the whole team sobbing with grief), but maintaining some distance also benefits the turtle. They have a greater chance of success when released if they are not conditioned to human presence, care, and affection.

"What was M like?" I asked.

"Sea turtles can get feisty—they should be able to whoop you pretty soundly, but M was the chillest turtle I have ever worked with."

M's story is from the first decade of the turtle's life, during which she had already endured extensive trauma and healing. Green sea turtles can live many decades, and because of their resilience Jeannie doesn't doubt that M will too. In 2015, two years after M's initial rescue, she was released into the Atlantic with great celebration. Fans and symbolic "adopters" who helped fund M's care grinned as they watched her return home to the ocean. All those folks on the beach that day have a turtle story, too, that they are unlikely to ever forget.

When I asked Jeannie if the tag could provide any updates on her success back in the wild, Jeannie replied, "M may still be tagged but she would have to be (temporarily) recaptured for us to know for sure how she's doing. We do often hear about recaptures of former patients, but we don't have any reports for M at this time. My personal rule is that any turtle we release does awesome and lives their best life!"

Rescuing and rehabilitating turtles requires resilience on the part of both the human and the beyond-human beings.

"So, why turtles in the first place?" I asked.

"Turtles kind of chose me!"

The choosing happened when Jeannie was on a spring break vacation in college with friends in Galveston, Texas. After they toured the National Marine Fisheries Service, she called home and told her family, "I'm either getting a job tomorrow, or I'm going to jail." The next day she returned to the property without a tour guide.

"I'm here to help," she said.

They took her up on her offer and she left that week with plans to return for a summer internship.

M's story is now one of hundreds for Jeannie, who continued to share turtle stories about other individuals she has known and distantly loved—some she helped to heal and others she couldn't, no matter how hard she and her team tried. When you seek turtle stories, you find turtle stories, and they don't stop rolling in!

✳ ✳ ✳

Turtles and tortoises have been described in the literature as "the most vulnerable animals alive."[6] After all, they face every threat a conservationist can conjure, from habitat loss to poaching to pollution to climate change. Yet, they also have "a smile that projects the wisdom of the earth"[7] and are "strong animals that keep secrets inside their shells."[8]

When my storytelling friends shared the one word they would use to describe turtles, I got responses like:

"Oh boy. That's hard."

And, "Other than *awesome?!*"

And, "Just *one?!*"

Responses included: *adorable* (of course), *threatened, equanimous, patient, gentle, old, determined,* and *resilient beyond words.*

It makes me wonder: What of the turtle's human stories? Did Curly feel some semblance of fear as he struggled, wedged between the rock and the pane of glass? What did the desert tortoise think about sharing his cave with a snoozing biologist? How often had M encountered another human between hatching and her harrowing beach rescue? Did the hawksbill female find the bioluminescent algae as magical to experience as Rachael did?

For my own turtle story, I spent two years photographing and taking notes on every eastern box turtle I encountered at the Clifton Institute, a northern Virginia nature preserve and nonprofit where I worked for a few years. I encountered twenty-one turtles, most of them in the summer. Based on the size and texture of each dome-like carapace, I estimated that a few of the individuals were more than thirty years old. Usually, the summer campers I accompanied spotted the critters before I did. Kids are closer to the ground where boxies roam and tend to have keener senses for spotting the subtle movements of wildlife. The reactions from children upon discovering a box turtle varied some but were always filled with awe.

"Dude, his neck is super–far out."

"It's a giraffe turtle, guys!"

Herpetologist Archie Carr once wrote, "In disposition box turtles also vary widely,"[9] and I certainly agree. Each one had a distinct personality, from shy to feisty. Some hissed and closed the hinge that gives box turtles their name, while others looked at us, curious and unafraid, indeed quite giraffe-like. Some peeked out from almost-closed shells and others took off through the leaf litter at a surprising speed. I loved to observe the variation in patterns on each turtle's shell. They ranged from black to yellow in color; some scutes (the individual "scales" on the shell) had ridges and some were smooth. My favorite turtles had bright orange neck skin and sweet brown eyes. We guessed their sexes by inspecting the plastron to see if it was concave or flat. (Males have a slightly more concave plastron so they can mount females.) Because of the pictures I took of each individual, I don't believe I ever encountered the same turtle twice, and that's pretty amazing considering that they are listed as vulnerable by the International Union for Conservation of Nature (IUCN). Many scientists are concerned about their declining populations.

My turtle story continues in *kurmasana*, turtle—or tortoise—pose. "This pose is sacred to a yogi," wrote B.K.S. Iyengar.[10] That's *my* turtle word: *sacred.* In kurmasana, I sit on the ground with my legs spread wide and fold forward as I slide my hands underneath my knees, along the sacred earth. It is challenging, but there are myriad tricks to make the pose more accessible. If viewed from above, I imagine I do look like a turtle, or at least the way kids draw cartoon turtles, minus the inevitable U-shaped tail: A head and four limbs stick out at all the right points from the shell created by my torso dutifully following the rules of gravity. There is also a version in which I bend my knees and bring the soles of my feet toward each other. It looks less turtle-y from above, but it feels properly *kurma.* I prefer the restorative version of kurmasana. In it, the heaviness of the earth on my back, left there by muskrat, provides a place for Skywoman to dance.

Kurmasana is grounding and comforting to me. The pose, wrote Iyengar, may refresh us "as though one had woken up from a long, undisturbed sleep."[11] Or a season of brumation. At autumn's end, I mourn the disappearance of turtles, and hear Michael Scott from *The Office* scream, "Where are the turtles?" They are headed into the earth's embrace.

Brumation is a period of dormancy, like hibernation, during which an organism becomes physically inactive. It is an adaptive strategy, used by some cold-blooded animals like reptiles and amphibians to survive cold temperatures. Freshwater turtles bury themselves in the mud at the bottom of the pond. Box turtles burrow into the soil and leaf litter. Anthony L. Rose wrote of the process, "When Lolita [the tortoise] dug in each winter she reentered the womb-grave of our mother, turned cold, and became again the earth. Buried alive for three months, she resurrected in spring. And in her brain, reverence for the transcendence was fixed. Would that it were so for us, warm-blooded scientists, terrified of the cold, the dark quiet earth."[12]

Like brumation, restorative yoga is a style of asana in which poses are held for longer periods of time, and supported by props (bolsters, blocks, straps, chairs, pillows, blankets, tree stumps, etc.) to facilitate comfort and relaxation. My human-and-herpetofauna-inclusive definition of brumation is a state of productive inactivity in a cozy spot during cold weather. For a turtle, in the mucky bottom of a lake. For a human, that cozy spot can be a yoga mat (or rug, or bed, or soft patch of moss) surrounded by blankets and pillows. Brumation, simply put, is what allows us all to survive. Without it, some animals wouldn't make it through the winter; and without the physiological and mental benefits of allowing our bodies productive relaxation, human life is a bit more of a struggle. Brumation restores us.

To brumate, we aim for the general shape of kurmasana, using props to support our torso and limbs to relieve the strain. Sitting on the corner of a folded blanket, I get a head start into my forward fold like Jeff's young terrapin trio. When the strain of the straddle is too great for the backs of my legs, I place foam blocks, rolled blankets, or pillows under my knees and lay my arms over them, piling more blankets between them for cushion and comfort. The props do not detract from the body making the shape of a turtle; in fact, they enhance it. We can drape blankets over our backs and pull the edges up over our heads when we desire darkness, quiet, and insulation from the world. But is this what we get? Not always. Our worries and to-do lists follow us under the blanket and "into the shell," amplified by the absence of sensory distraction.

The discussion about turtles in the yoga world is often linked to pratyahara, one of the other eight limbs of yoga—in addition to asana—that refers to the internalization or withdrawal of the senses like "a tortoise draws back into its shell," according to verse 2:58 of the *Bhagavad Gita*.[13] The text draws a direct comparison to the animal and suggests that when we do the same with our senses, our insight is clearest. Additionally, in yoga asana, forward-bending poses are said to promote introspection or turning inward.

Yet, pratyahara is inconsistent with my own observations of turtles and tortoises, and the stories shared to me by others about them. Turtles do not withdraw inside their 220-million-year-old shells.[14] Not all turtles can go inside their shells. For example, sea turtles are unable to retract their heads or flippers, but that doesn't render the shell useless—it is still an integral part of the turtle's anatomy that protects their inner organs. For those turtles who do "retreat into their shells," this is simply another way of being their wise, ancient selves in the world instead of leaving it behind. The pratyahara comparison is appropriate during brumation, but what about the other nine months of the year? If they were all so often withdrawn, if they didn't engage with the world, people wouldn't have the opportunity to connect with them as the abundance of turtle stories demonstrates.

In fact, turtles *are* their shells. It's like another human telling you to withdraw into your body. Impossible physically; but, oddly enough, this is what yoga and pratyahara require of us in other ways. Turtles don't make homes inside their shells. They *are* their homes. Carrying the mud and the mountain on their backs, turtles are our home too. Joseph Bruchac wrote, "This earth itself is as alive as that great turtle which supports us on its back."[15] In this way, turtles guide us toward the realization that we are the sacred animals we seek. We search for home, but we are already there, either with giant, barnacle-encrusted shells or spindly, internal rib cages.

To be clear, my intention is not to disrespect the idea of pratyahara or argue that it is not a concept worthy of study. In our restorative asana practice we seek to withdraw our attention from external distractions and focus on the experiences within our own bodies. We must let our senses, like our bodies, rest.[16] By burrowing into the embrace of the earth and minimizing sensory input for a few minutes or months, we emerge more open to the world around us, so that our "intuitive intelligence can function usefully and in a worthwhile manner."[17] Instead of stretching and strengthening as in an active asana practice, restorative kurmasana creates opening in the legs and hips like turtles open us up to the world instead of encouraging us to turn away from it. I simply suggest we pause before we associate pratyahara with turtles and tortoises, lest we limit the ways in which we can better understand them.

There are approximately 340 species in the order Testudines,[18] to which turtles and tortoises belong, and there is much variation within and among species. Turtles are not always slow, and they are rarely green like in cartoon depictions and children's illustrations. What else are we missing? Turtle joy? Turtle grief? Some scientists might be quick to say that these are the types of experiences of other animals that we will never understand, but anthropologist and animal advocate Barbara J. King said that to find turtle grief we must look for it. She wrote of a male sea turtle seeming to mourn a picture of a dead female, of a tortoise who helped another tortoise right himself, and of a soft-shelled turtle named Pigface who played basketball at the National Zoo.[19] Once we have established that turtles are about more than withdrawing into their shells, we can get to know these critters beyond their stereotypical portrayals and beyond our own perceptions of who turtles are.

For this reason, turtles are the resolution to the friction I used to sense regarding the idea of *wild asana*. It used to feel like a contradiction that we should be focused internally on our own bodies and minds, while simultaneously remaining aware of—even immersed in—the natural world around us in all its spiral-shelled, leather-egged glory. Turtles do both. With the resilience of the turtle and periodic brumation, we are better able to shoulder the weight of this sacred world instead of running from it—or worse, hiding from it.

Practice
RESTORATIVE BRUMATION YOGA

Brumate like a turtle. It's good for your survival! Surrender to the "womb-grave of our mother"[20] and drape a weighted bolster or blanket over your back. According to Judith Hanson Lasater, there are four requirements for the ideal restorative yoga experience:

1. Stillness: A brumating animal becomes lethargic and rarely, if ever, moves. Make yourself comfortable, sink into the support of your props, and rest without moving.

2. Darkness: Animals brumate in places where little light penetrates, including burrows, caves in the desert, and under rocks, leaf litter, or water. Dim the lights and close your eyes. Put a blanket over your head to experience what it's like to be part shell.

3. Warmth: Brumating animals' body temperatures are determined by their surroundings, so during the coldest months they seek out insulated places to ensure they will not freeze. Wear thick socks and a cozy wool sweater.

4. Silence: Brumating animals' heartbeats, breathing, and digestion slow way down. Practice alone in a quiet, secluded space.

After you unhinge your plastron and reemerge in the world, call a friend to share an animal story of your own. Talk about an encounter with a fellow being. Text them and say, "I want to share with you about the time that I saw a cloud of dragonflies. . . ." Tweet your story. Tik-Tok it. Paint your story and hang it on the wall for others to see. Dance it. Ask someone else their turtle story, or that of any sacred animal. See where the conversation takes you.

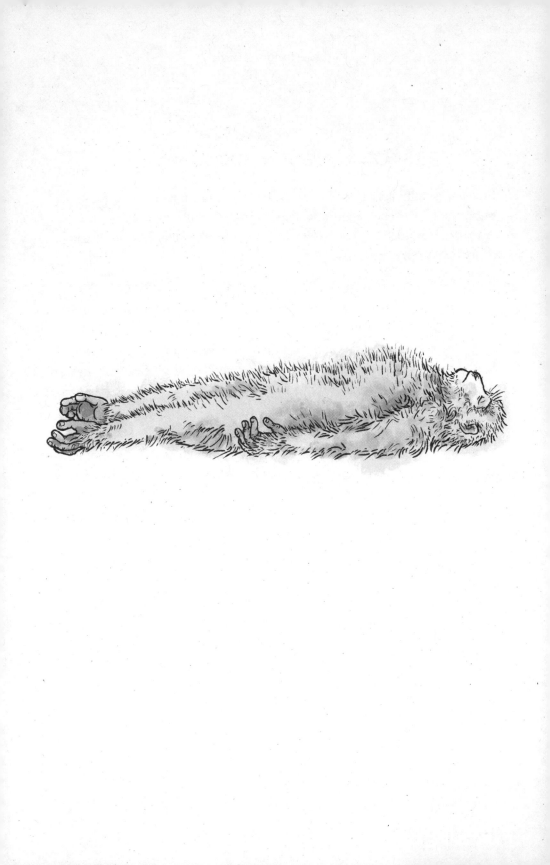

Chapter 13

SAVA—CORPSE

The farmer plucked a watermelon from the vine and cut it into chunks with a machete. We sat in the garden surrounded by forest, munching on the fruit as the juice trickled down and dripped off our elbows into the dirt. I was in Sulawesi, conducting anthropological research on the wildlife consumption of human-cultivated foods. I chatted with farmers in between greedy bites of the snack that was grown in the ground upon which I squatted. I wasn't the only primate around here who coveted the fruit, although the farmers shared with me willingly.

"Be careful," they warned, snickering.

"Why?" I asked.

"Later you're really going to have to pee!"

As our laughter died down, the tone of the conversation changed.

"Those monkeys, if they die," said one of the farmers, "you can't find the carcass, you know? You can't find it anywhere!"

"The body?" I asked, double-checking my understanding of a new-to-me Indonesian word.

Corpse.

Sava, in Sanskrit.

"Yeah. For example, if someone says, 'I saw a dead monkey there yesterday,' and then you go look for it, you can't find it! Maybe a friend took it. Because if they die there's nothing that eats them!" he said.

By *friend* he meant another monkey, a term that farmers often used when referring to interactions between different individuals in the same social group. I had never heard anything about this before, and I didn't question him further.

We finished off the watermelon and it was time for my research partner, Amir, and I to leave for the day. I thanked the farmers for sharing a part of their harvest with me, stashed my notebook and pen, put on my helmet, and climbed onto the back of Amir's motorcycle. The route home began with a jarring couple of miles down a rocky trail on the way to the main road.

Although I was used to the brain-rattling ride by now, it occurred to me that I would never survive the trip home without peeing first. I suddenly needed to go so badly that I panicked. This close to the garden, I would have to walk some distance to find a private place. In fact, I had to walk back past the group of all-male farmers on my quest for the perfect pee spot. I passed alone, with a sheepish grin on my face, waving for comic effect. They all knew exactly where I was going and exploded with laughter.

I walked until I could no longer hear them. As soon as I started to empty my bladder, I heard rustling vegetation. Two cows appeared and stared at me until I pulled up my pants. I stood, and they lumbered off in the direction they came.

That problem solved, I replayed a single question in my mind the whole way home: Why don't people find the bodies of dead monkeys? I asked Amir if he ever saw one and he said no. Apparently this was already a topic of discussion among the locals, because he told me that Pak Haro, the "monkey whisperer" who has been following the animals in their forest habitat for over thirty years, has never seen the body of a dead monkey.

Primates are social, so we should expect an individual's death to have some effect on the still-living animals. Most of what we know about dead monkeys is from anecdotal reports about how surviving group members deal with death, often of an infant. A wide range of behaviors has been observed in this scenario, from others ignoring the corpse to a mother carrying her dead infant for days as the body rots.[1] Occasionally, researchers find dead adult monkeys as they follow the groups they study. One research team aimed a camera trap at a golden snub-nosed monkey carcass to see who scavenged the body (answer: a civet, a black bear, crows, and rats).[2] Another recorded the deaths of howler monkeys that succumbed to yellow fever in Argentina.[3] There is even a monkey cemetery at a wildlife sanctuary in Ghana where dead monkeys who die of "old age or accidents" enjoy a ceremonial burial by local human residents.[4] The corpses, somewhere, and sometimes, are discovered.

A week later, in the home of another farmer, I received the same question in a voice full of genuine curiosity. "Dead dogs are eaten by pigs and dead pigs are eaten by dogs, but what happens to dead monkeys? I've never seen a body!" he explained.

Another man chimed in. "Maybe they take away the bodies. Maybe they have a place for that like people do, like in a cave or a hole in a tree."

Like a grave, I thought but didn't say.

"Maybe they eat the body. Because no other animal would eat a dead monkey." Someone added the suggestion that other animals, like people, don't eat monkeys because it is forbidden by Islam.

What happens to the corpse of a monkey? I was excited to discuss this question with my primatology friends and fellow researchers, the ones who spent most of their time following the monkeys and observing their behavior. I, on the other hand, instead spent a lot of time with people and plants, while camera traps recorded the monkey business. My friends reacted as if I was silly for entertaining these ideas and offered logical explanations for why no one ever finds the carcass of a dead monkey. The body decomposes quickly in the tropical climate. A dying monkey intentionally separates itself from the group. Dogs *do* eat them. . . .

So, my conversations with the farmers weren't rigorously scientific, but they were still productive. By considering behaviors outside the realm of our academic understanding, we learn more about the community that shares the forest with the monkeys. We understand a little more intimately the ways in which farmers perceive their primate neighbors, and we experiment with other ways of knowing beyond-human beings. I refuse to believe that's not worth something; so, while I can't tell you where local monkeys go to practice their final savasana, I *can* tell you where to find the world's best watermelon.

※ ※ ※

Savasana, also known as corpse pose, is practiced lying on the back with the spine in alignment, the feet relaxed as the legs rotate externally, and the palms facing up with fingers gently curled. When I prepare for savasana I fidget and wriggle until the back of my head is flat on the floor and my arms rest at the preferred angle to my supine body. I relax the muscles in my face for the first time that day, maybe for the first time this life. Author Lyanda Lynn Haupt writes that savasana is "a reminder that the world can do very well without us for a short time, and will eventually do very well without us altogether."[5]

Benefits of savasana may include, most notably, a positive effect on the parasympathetic nervous system that allows our bodies to rest and digest. According to expert yoga teacher Judith Hanson Lasater, this one pose has the potential, when practiced regularly, to refresh our mood, reduce stress and anxiety, slow the effects of aging on the body, improve sleep, and reduce blood sugar and cholesterol levels.[6] As the end of savasana signals the transition away from our asana practice, death (of the physical body or, instead, a more metaphorical kind) is one of the most important transitions we and other beings experience.

Savasana need not represent only the human corpse. The mysterious exception of some monkeys aside, animal bodies of all shapes and sizes litter the earth in various stages of death and decomposition. We observe many more beyond-human corpses in our lifetime than human ones. We are destroyers. Sometimes we create a corpse with our shoe, a tire, or even with our own hand. I have slapped countless mosquitoes (on purpose), accidentally rolled the wheel of a gate over the soft body of an anole, and hit a raccoon, a rabbit, and a mourning dove with my car. That last one was the most devastating. I could no longer see the road to drive as I wailed, "I'm so sorry!" on repeat as my mind replayed the spray of feathers near my front right tire on an endless loop. I called my brand-new boyfriend, sobbing uncontrollably. (He married me anyway, bless his heart!) If suffering inevitably exists, as the first Noble Truth in Buddhism advises, then we must accept that we cannot exist without harming other beings. All we can do is try our best to limit the harm.

On my commute one morning, from my suburban home to a more rural county to the west, I counted five carcasses (and nearly missed a live squirrel). There were two deer, a red fox, a Canada goose, and a raccoon. With each corpse I passed I wondered how many more animals were hit and had crawled just far enough away from the grimy medians and gravel-strewn shoulders to die under shrouds of grass. I hoped their lives, no less valuable than mine, were long and their suffering short. The bloated doe on which the crow fed had fawns to carry and birth, nurse, and groom. She had shrubs to browse, hunters to hide from, and coyotes to avoid. She had sunsets to watch with eyes like dark pools from her bed of stomped-down sumac and little bluestem. Her purpose in life could not have been to teach a driver not to speed.

I knew how deeply I loved my husband when I saw his reaction to a snake run over by another car, as we traveled Skyline Drive in Shenandoah National Park. It happened so fast. I doubt they meant to hit the snake, though I know some drivers do aim for wildlife in this horrific manner. The road was twisty and turny, and we were passing another car headed in the opposite direction as the snake chose that second to cross the road. We watched the tire of the car hit the snake. Then we watched the snake thrash around helplessly. Vishu squeezed his eyes shut and pounded a tight fist against his thigh as a sharp sigh escaped his lips. I might yell and point when I realize what is about to happen, but when it does, I am frozen. The expression on my face is blank. I shut down except for my mind in which the scene replays over and over for minutes, maybe hours, maybe days with fading frequency. But Vishu's reaction was visceral and involuntary. The grief and care for a creature he never knew was written all over his face.

Yet, even after death there is life. I first suspected there was magic in savasana when I wiggled my fingers and they tingled with pleasure, gratitude, and remembrance that they were indeed a part of this body—and very much alive. An arguably more "animal" variation of this pose is the side-lying version in which the head is supported by blankets and the knees hugged in toward the chest. With my body in this position, I feel curled up, cozy, and safe. Many teachers transition their students out of savasana with a minute or two of side-lying before they sit up again. In this way, we move from corpse to the fetal position. We are reborn. Our eyes flutter open, we fold our hands in front of our hearts, and we stumble out of savasana and back into the world. Into our cars to sit in traffic.

✳ ✳ ✳

Indeed, there is life from beyond-human beings who are killed in the road—just ask a vulture.

An old vulture king named Jatayu is the unsung hero of the Hindu epic the Ramayana. He was the first friendly critter to appear in some retellings,[7] and the guardian of Prince Rama and Princess Sita's hut during their exile in the forest. Jatayu witnessed Sita's kidnapping by the demon Ravana, who then cut off his wing with a sword. "The bird fell to the ground . . . doing marvelous feats of courage," after which Rama and his brother Lakshmana found Jatayu earthbound and bleeding. Before he succumbed to his injuries, Jatayu explained that Ravana took Sita to the south, "crying as piteously as an osprey."[8]

As Rama prepared for the funeral rituals, Lakshmana questioned why he treated a mere bird with such respect. Rama defended Jatayu, explaining that since the bird acted with such courage and compassion, of course they should cremate the creature who helped them. "The tender-hearted and compassionate [Rama], who shows mercy even on the undeserving bestowed upon a vulture, an unclean, flesh-eating bird."[9]

Jatayu was not so undeserving and unclean. Vultures alive today are a far osprey's cry from these negative descriptors. In fact, they are built, inside and out, for maintaining cleanliness for themselves and the ecosystems they inhabit. Their bald heads prevent corpse goo from rotting in their feathers, and some have see-through, pervious nostrils that allow for easy unclogging. Vultures also have digestive tracts with pH measurements meant to destroy microscopic organisms that cause infection, thus reducing the spread of disease.[10] They intentionally excrete uric acid on their own legs to kill germs and bacteria. Around the world, the decline in vulture populations has led to an increase in feral dogs and rats who spread infectious diseases to people, livestock, and wildlife. Scavengers play essential roles in entire communities of plants and animals upon which humans rely, as they aid in the decomposition process. Vultures are as deserving of our appreciation as the staff busing tables in restaurants, and the workers collecting from our curbs the garbage we have the luxury to forget about before we've double-tied the trash bag closed.

Vultures are also culturally important to many communities, and even play a role in funeral practices in Persian Zoroastrian and Tibetan Buddhist traditions.[11] In the Upper Mustang region of Nepal, the practice is called *jhator*, or sky burial. When a person dies, their corpse is brought to an exposed area. Then vultures are attracted to the spot with prayers and bells and invited to consume the body. In doing so, they take the deceased person's soul to the next phase in the wheel of life.[12]

The battle that eventually occurred on the island of Lanka, to free Sita, is often described as the victory of good over evil. Yet, in the Ramayana as in ecology, everything is interconnected, and creatures are not always what they seem. For example, this "villain" was not always the bad guy. In many versions of the story, Ravana captured Sita in retaliation for a previous incident during which Rama injured his sister. Scorpions do not sting out of malice, and snakes are no longer the devil as soon as you know them as individual beings. Vultures are not unclean or undeserving of our respect. It turns out that the "good versus evil" dichotomy is about as useful as "human versus animal."

At first, the Ramayana is an intimidating story to learn. I read every retelling I can get my hands on, and plot points still elude me—especially because they vary from version to version. But connecting asana to stories like the Ramayana and other teachings from South Asia is an important component of efforts to decolonize yoga, a practice that here in the West has become diluted and polluted with tight pants, body shaming, toxic positivity, spiritual bypassing, cultural appropriation, and more. By honoring the roots of yoga, we "preserve the heart and soul of this powerful practice for future generations," according to Susanna Barkataki.[13] It is challenging work that requires a commitment to non-harming, truth-telling, and deep listening, but it is our responsibility.

There is no doubt that Sita would not have been rescued as quickly if Jatayu had not sacrificed his life. Ravana would have kidnapped her entirely undetected and unchallenged. He visited the hut in a flying chariot, leaving no footprints for Rama to follow. Only a creature capable of high-altitude flight could have intervened as Jatayu did. Vultures are heroes. Channeling Jatayu in savasana, we believe that we have done everything we can with what we have. We know that we have done our best. We're confident that we have given all of ourselves, but only for what we believe in and for those we love, with all our being. We've fulfilled our purpose for this hour or this day or this life, and for now, we rest.

✳ ✳ ✳

I knew a few turkey vultures, TUVUs for short, when I volunteered at the Rocky Mountain Raptor Program, a rehabilitation center for birds of prey in Fort Collins, Colorado. They were wily things with curious stares and tangible personalities. (Vulturalities? Animalities?) There was also the captive black vulture at the Tallahassee Museum who hopped along the ground on white legs, following me around the edge of its chain-link enclosure like a dog wanting to play. While working as a zoo educator at Busch Gardens in college, I watched countless tourists speed past the wise-eyed and handsome white-backed vulture on their way to the snoozing lion.

"What, really, is death?" I should have asked them all.

Buddhist monks meditate on death in cemeteries; I open my guide to *Mammal Tracks & Sign* and turn to the section titled "Interpreting Prey Remains."[14] Through photographs of suffocated fawns, fur-plucked calves, brainless fish, half-buried elk, and goats dangling from tree-branch caches, I learn about the various ways North American beyond-human hunters ambush, kill, and consume their prey. With every small gasp at the sight of a mangled corpse I imagine a predator plump and satiated, her muzzle stained with blood. In her book *Animal Intimacies: Interspecies Relatedness in India's Central Himalayas*, Radhika Govindrajan writes:

> There were some animals that I came to know mostly or almost entirely
> through their material and immaterial traces—green bear scat, covered in
> loud, iridescent flies, lying in the middle of a mountain path; the half-eaten
> bovine carcass that a leopard had carefully dragged to the side of the road;
> the loud squeals and grunts of a particular group of wild boar who made
> regular, nocturnal visits to the fields directly below a house I lived in. These
> traces were visceral evocations of the animals who left them.[15]

On the hiking trails of the nature preserve where I worked in Virginia, my students and I were lucky to find scat and to experience the sounds and smells of the living. But even when those visceral evocations came instead from a corpse, or a part of one, there was life. There were carrion beetles and maggots and fungi to inspect. There were vultures riding the thermals high above our heads. There was a predator no longer hungry.

One evening, on a hike with a group of eighteen young scouts, we found ourselves crowded around a small, lifeless body in the middle of the trail.

"I think it's a mole," said one of the children.

It wasn't a mole, but the species wasn't important. Its death was. We leaned in for a closer look. The kids were mostly quiet. A boy poked at the body gingerly with his crooked hiking stick. Nothing happened.

Of course, they eventually started to ask, "What happened to it?"

Of course, I didn't know. We could all only guess.

We talked briefly about who might eat the "mole," the process of decomposition, and the recycling of nutrients, but none of that seemed important. The only thing we knew for sure was that things die. And now that dead "mole" will provide life for something else.

"It makes me feel kind of sad," said one of the youngest boys.

And with that we walked away. A little quieter, a little more thoughtful. But confident knowing that—mole or vole, mature tulip poplar or microscopic moss piglet—the forest and its creatures will, in some way, go on existing in our absence.

Yoga teachers trained in trauma-informed programs learn to refer to savasana as a "final relaxation" to avoid the word *corpse*. But death is less of a "final relaxation" and more of a continuation of life in a different form. It is not a moment in time, but a transition. Think decomposition. When a tree dies there are different categories of deadness like "dead spongy," "dead soft," and "dead fallen."[16] Instead of becoming more dead with time, it becomes more alive. Eventually, a dead tree is not dead at all—it's just dirt. Existence on this earth requires us to live with, die with, and even decompose with other animals.[17] And that is where I'm happy. Would you rather be enlightened and released from the cycle of death and rebirth or remain on this beautiful planet with our fellow animals? Maybe it's win-win. Life comes from death. This is not the end.

Practice

"LOVINGKINDNESS BEYOND THE HUMAN" MEDITATION

Reflecting on many variations of existing lovingkindness meditations, I started to wonder why we are limited to primarily wishing lovingkindness for ourselves and other humans (until the end, when all beings everywhere are included). So, I created my own version of this popular meditation, flipping the order of the traditional practice so it starts with all beings everywhere, ends with ourselves, and includes more beyond-human beings along the way. (Since no one can read a book and meditate at the same time, visit my website, www .alisonzak.com, for an audio version of this meditation.) Sit outside for this one, right on the earth!

To begin, make sure you are seated comfortably. Relax the muscles in your face. Relax your jaw. Relax your hips. Release any gripping in the legs. Your hands can rest in your lap or on your knees. Become aware of the place where your body meets the earth. Imagine yourself physically rooted into the earth and smile as her support simultaneously grounds and uplifts you. Close your eyes and notice your breath. Observe each inhale and each exhale. Remember the present moment.

Now, imagine earth and all the beings on our amazing planet. If you're already feeling overwhelmed or challenged, you're doing it right. This shouldn't be easy! We are going to cultivate lovingkindness for the earth and all its living beings with three intentions. You can repeat them in your mind, say them aloud, or simply concentrate on their meaning.

May all beings and the earth be healthy and safe.

May all beings and the earth feel happy and at peace.

May all beings and the earth be free from suffering.

Now imagine a nonhuman being, or group of beings, with which you have a difficult, complex, or conflicting relationship. A mosquito that bit you, your neighbor's dog who barks too often, or even an animal whose products you use or consume. We will wish them lovingkindness, too.

May you be healthy and safe.

May you feel happy and at peace.

May you be free from suffering.

Imagine a neutral nonhuman being. A creature you neither love nor struggle to love. A cow you drove past in your car, the grass cushioning your bum, a goose on the sidewalk....

May you be healthy and safe.

May you feel happy and at peace.

May you be free from suffering.

Now, recall a nonhuman being that you love. The tree you used to climb in your parents' backyard, a beloved pet . . . this one's easy!

May you be healthy and safe.

May you feel happy and at peace.

May you be free from suffering.

Finally, bring your attention to yourself. For some people, this is the hardest part of all, but really wish this for yourself.

May I be healthy and safe.

May I feel happy and at peace.

May I be free from suffering.

If it feels strange to end with yourself, remember that "all beings and the earth" are not separate from ourselves. They are us. We are one. With your next inhale, receive a delicious breath from the earth. Exhale, and open your eyes.

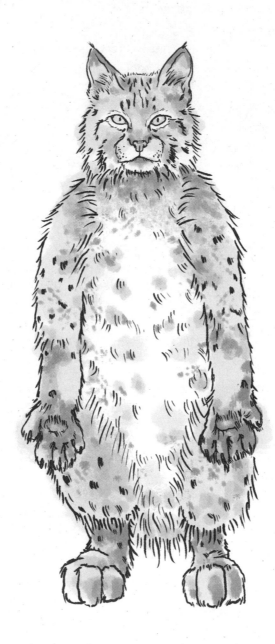

Conclusion

TADASANA—
MOUNTAIN POSE

Aldo Leopold, environmentalist and author of *A Sand County Almanac*, published an essay in 1949 titled "Thinking Like a Mountain."

But I don't think mountains think. I feel that they feel.

Leopold had to learn that the mountain needed grass and deer and wolves, but the mountain already knew. She could feel the tickle of the fish's fins, the silent whoosh of the eagle's wing, the pricking of the bobcat's claws in her soil, and the warmth from the body of the decomposing dove.

The green fire that Leopold watched fade from the eyes of the wolf mother he shot and killed not only dwells within the wolf and the mountain, but also burns deep inside our own hearts. The mountain feels our footsteps when we walk and our hearts beat when we lie down upon the earth. She feels that we are all connected, interdependent. From her perspective, we are all animals, and we are all the sacred same despite our celebrated differences.

Leopold also wrote, "Only the mountain has lived long enough to listen objectively to the howl of a wolf."[1]

But why would she want to? Mountains are not objective beings, and neither are we. I want to listen to the howl of a wolf and feel something. Fear, love, sorrow, joy—all of the holy above. I want to be anything but objective. I want to be alive and complex and ever-changing. I want to feel wild when I listen to wolves because the wild is within me.

If "wildness is the preservation of the world," as Henry David Thoreau wrote,[2] then being and feeling—instead of thinking—like a mountain will better help us discover the wild inside. Our wildness is not lost or gone or forgotten. It is temporarily unrealized.[3] Realizing it will be painfully simple and profoundly healing. Like breathing. Or watching the sun rise while watching the sunrise. It will be worth it.

This is not a quaint idea or friendly invitation; it is an urgent plea. Connecting with other animals in mindful and meaningful ways is our responsibility. It doesn't have to happen out in "pristine wilderness," in solitude, or under risky conditions like it did for the naturalists of yore. It happens in our homes and backyards and cities, with our families and communities, infused with our cultures. It can happen on our yoga mats, but it doesn't have to. There is never only one path or practice that leads to this worthy destination. Our goal does have to be Yoga, though, in its most universal sense, the yoking of ourselves to other beings and to nature in wild ways so that we can save each other and our earth.

Stand tall in mountain pose, *tadasana,* simultaneously rooted and rising tall. Ditch your yoga mat and let the grass tickle your skin. Don't only imagine rooting your feet into the earth . . . *do* it. Feel the dampness of the dirt. Let mosquitoes buzz around your face. Delight in ants dancing in the grass. Embody the pigeon, the snake, the cat, in form and in thought as you breathe your own animal breath and move your own animal body into shapes that revere your fellow creatures, yourself. Make your green fire fierce. Less thinking, more being and feeling. And more mountains, always more mountains.

Wild Asana
PRACTICE SEQUENCE

This short asana sequence includes poses named after mammals, birds, reptiles, insects, arachnids, and fish, domestic animals, wild animals, and those in between. As you move, reflect on how animals look, move, and behave to inspire your practice. The ultimate goal is to achieve Yoga—union—with beyond-human beings. To remember that we are animals and a part of nature too. Practice on a soft yet supportive surface such as a yoga mat, rug, blanket, or grass.

Note: Especially if you are new to yoga asana, practice these poses in a class led by an experienced teacher, listen to your own body, and never put yourself in any position that causes discomfort or pain. Many of the animal poses are challenging even for those who have been practicing for years. Remember that yoga is not about achieving a certain shape or comparing yourself to anyone else. It doesn't matter what the pose "should" look like—it only matters that you feel steady and comfortable in your animal body.

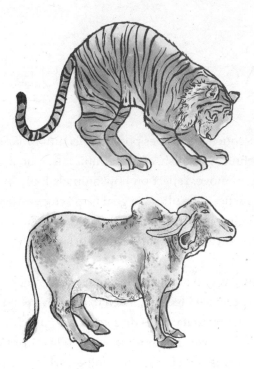

CAT/COW FLOW

Begin on your hands and knees. Position your hands underneath your shoulders and your knees underneath your hips. You can add a folded blanket under the knees for some extra cushion. Flex your spine, dropping your belly button toward the floor and gazing up. Then arch your spine and tuck your chin to your chest as you raise your mid-back toward the ceiling. Feel your pelvis tilting forward and back as you flow through cat and cow shapes. You can also choose to flex and arch your spine while seated on the edge of a chair. Feel your spine elongating and contracting. Partner with your breath, inhaling for cow, exhaling for cat, until sufficiently quadrupedal. Return to a neutral, divine spine.

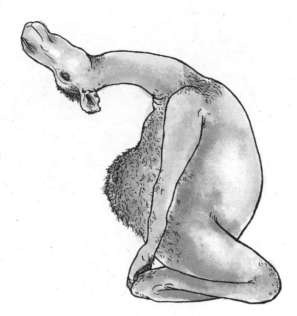

USTRASANA—CAMEL POSE

Come up onto your knees and reach your hands toward the sky. Keep your toes curled under or place the tops of your feet flat onto the floor. Arch your back, release your right hand to behind your right hip with the fingers pointing down. To bend more deeply, reach your hand past your hip toward your right heel. Open through your heart as you bend, letting your chest float subtly toward the sky. Use a foam block or knitting needle as an arm-extender that lands on the floor next to your heel. Repeat on the left side. For a symmetrical, deep backbend, reach both hands to the backs of your hips, then toward your heels at the same time. For a gentler version, sit on the edge of a chair, reach your hands toward the sky, lift and open your chest, and grasp the chair back with your hands (one at a time or together), inching your hands down until you feel comfortably camel. Keep lifting the chest up and open, and protect your neck by keeping the muscles engaged and staying in control of the weight of your head.

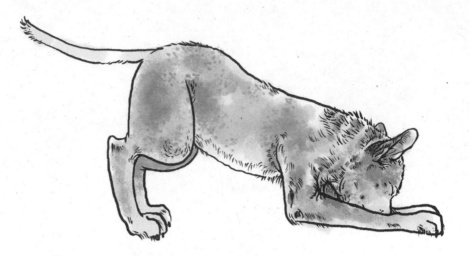

UTTANA SHISHOSANA
(ALSO KNOWN AS PUPPY POSE)

From kneeling on all fours, keep your hips where they are and walk your hands forward about two feet. Sink your chest toward the earth and reach your arms out in front of you. Rest your forehead on the floor or a block. Play-bow like a puppy. Wag your tail, moving your spine in a gentle side stretch laterally in both directions. Walk your hands back so they're straight under your shoulders, as you return to kneel like a table with a neutral spine. From a chair, walk your feet wide and fold forward from the hips, bending all the way down and walking your hands away from you along the ground.

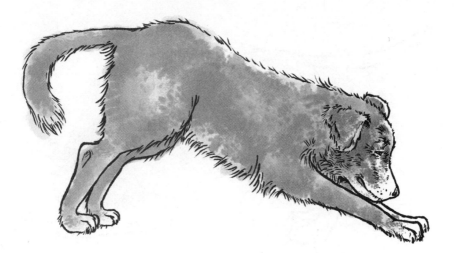

ADHO MUKHA SVANASANA—
DOWNWARD-FACING DOG POSE

From kneeling, move your hands one pawprint forward. Curl your toes under and lift your hips. Bend your knees so you can reach your spine long as you relax your neck and let your head dangle. Engage the muscles in the backs of your legs by imagining your heels reaching toward the floor. Press into all ten fingertips, keep your elbows softly bent, and push up and out of your shoulders. To play with a gentler version, stand a few feet from the back of your chair, hinge from your hips and fold yourself into (roughly) a right angle as your hands grip the back of the chair. Slowly walk your feet away from the chair until you feel a stretch in your torso and the backs of your legs. Keep your knees bent any amount. Pedal your feet. Get "the zoomies." Howl out loud.

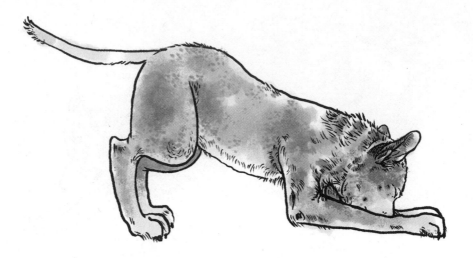

UTTANA SHISHOSANA
(ALSO KNOWN AS PUPPY POSE)

Bring your knees to the ground, a little wider than hip distance. Uncurl your toes. Guide your chest toward the floor and walk your hands forward, keeping your hips high. Place your forehead on the ground and reach your arms along the ground in front of you.

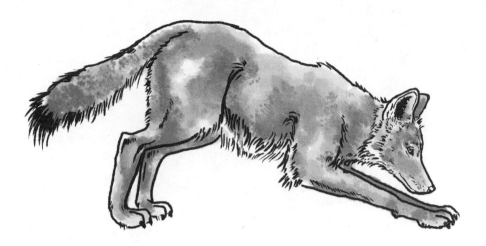

ADHO MUKHA SVANASANA—
DOWNWARD-FACING COYOTE POSE

Good dog. Come up again through a table position, move your hands forward a few inches, and lift your hips up into downward-facing coyote. Feel your spine stretching nice and long. Lift your right leg behind you. Keep your hips square toward the floor for a couple of breaths, then bend your right knee and open up your hips, pointing your right knee toward the sky. Reach your left heel closer to the floor. Then step your right foot between your hands, scooching it up in as many steps as needed. Drop your back knee onto a folded blanket for cushioning.

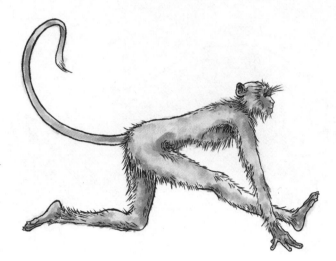

ARDHA HANUMANASANA— HALF-MONKEY SPLIT POSE

Flow from this low lunge to a half-split, straightening your front leg toward the front of your mat while your back knee remains bent. Shift your hips forward and backward, bending and straightening your right knee. Your hands can stay on the ground on either side of your right foot or walk back and forth along the floor as you move. You can also place your hands on foam blocks or thick books. The toes of your back foot can be curled or not. To practice "half-splits" with a chair, stand facing the side of the chair and place your right foot on the seat. Shift your hips back and forth, bending and straightening your right knee. Move with your breath, forward on the inhale, backward on the exhale. This flow helps to stretch the legs and open the hips in preparation for hanumanasana.

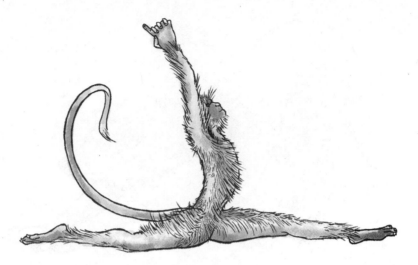

HANUMANASANA—MONKEY SPLIT POSE

Pause in your lunge with your right foot in between your hands and your left leg long behind you (knee on a blanket on the ground). Slide your right foot forward and your left foot back by curling your toes and moving inch by inch. Sink your primate hips toward the floor and onto a stack of blocks, pile of books, tower of pillows, or the seat of a chair. From wherever you land, savor the sensation of your feet reaching energetically in opposite directions. Explore the idea of lifting your hands and reaching them toward the sky as your hips ground down. *Jai Hanuman.* Mindfully, inch out of the split.

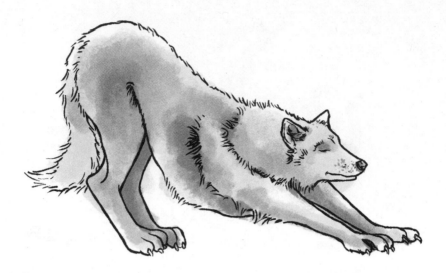

ADHO MUKHA SVANASANA— DOWNWARD-FACING WOLF POSE

Come back through a table position, move the hands forward a few inches, and lift the hips up into downward-facing wolf. Remember to relax your head and neck and let your knees bend. Lift your left leg behind you. Keep your hips square toward the floor for a couple of breaths, then bend your left knee and open up your hips, pointing your left knee toward the sky. Reach your right heel closer to the floor. Then step your left foot between your hands and drop your back knee onto the blanket.

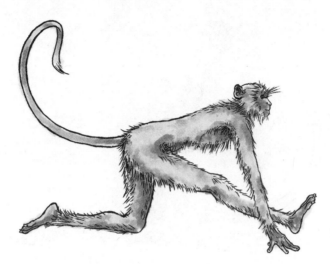

ARDHA HANUMANASANA— HALF-MONKEY SPLIT POSE

Flow again from a low lunge to a half-split, shifting your hips back and forth, bending and straightening your left knee. Use your props as needed and remember to move with your breath, inhaling to a low lunge and exhaling into a half-split.

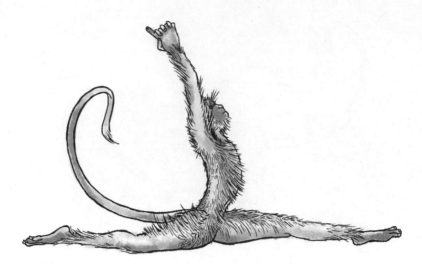

HANUMANASANA—MONKEY SPLIT POSE

Pause in your low lunge with your left foot in between your hands. Slide your left foot forward and your right foot back, inching yourself only to the edge of your comfort. Guide your hips toward the floor and onto the props of your choice. Notice how your body might feel differently on this side compared to the other. Inch out of the split with devotion to your monkey mind.

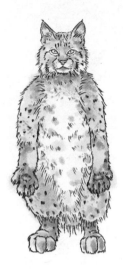

TADASANA—MOUNTAIN POSE

Stand tall, planting your feet firmly onto the earth. Experiment with the distance between your feet (hip-width, wider-than-hips, inner edges of the feet touching) and find stability. Stand in tadasana with your spine tall. For a seated version, sit on the edge of a chair. Root down through your feet and rise up from the top of your head. Let your arms hang naturally at your sides. Tuck your chin slightly and gaze down a few feet in front of you on the floor. Notice how it feels to root and rise at the same time with all your spine's natural curves. You are immersed in fierce, green, fauna fire.

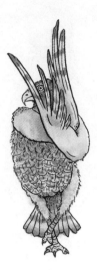

GARUDASANA—EAGLE POSE

Shift your weight into your left leg. Curl your right foot around the outside of your left calf. Your toes can also come to the floor on the outside of your opposite foot or onto a block. Bend both knees any amount to drop your hips and allow for entanglement. Repeat on the opposite side. Return to standing. Then, bend both arms and cross your left elbow on top of your right and intertwine your forearms and hands. You can bring the backs of your palms toward each other, or for a deeper shoulder stretch, hook your bottom fingers into your top palm. Repeat on the other side. Practice the leg and arm components of the pose separately, until you feel ready to combine them. Whichever leg is on top, your arm on that same side goes underneath. Balance for a few breaths, then unwind yourself, surrendering. Shake it out and repeat on the other side. To practice garudasana from a chair, sit tall, cross your right thigh over your left, and squeeze your legs together. Give yourself a hug, then switch sides. Tangle and untangle.

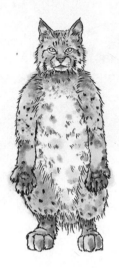

TADASANA—MOUNTAIN POSE

Shake out your limbs and stand again to feel like a mountain, noticing changes to your balance or sense of rootedness.

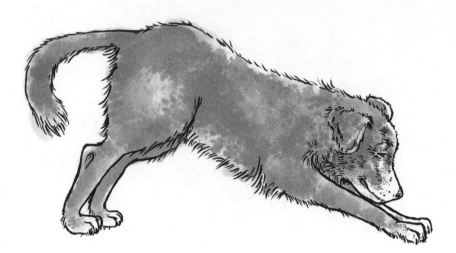

ADHO MUKHA SVANASANA— DOWNWARD-FACING DOG POSE

Fold in half at your hips, bend your knees, and place your hands on the floor (or onto blocks) underneath your shoulders. Step both feet backward. Lift your hips, relax your head, reach your heels toward the ground. Find stillness here. Not rest, but stillness.

The following two poses are especially challenging and optional. If firefly and scorpion pose are familiar to you and you can practice them confidently and safely, please do so. If not, return to adho mukha svanasana and playfully lift one foot as you hop up and down on the bottom foot to get the feel of balancing, even for a second, on your arms. Then skip to bhujangasana.

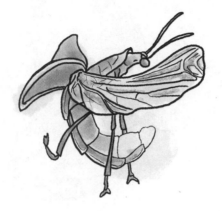

TITTIBHASANA—FIREFLY POSE

This pose requires significant core and arm strength, open hips and hamstrings, and warmed-up wrists. Come into a squat, reach your arms around the backs of your calves and plant your palms on the ground with your fingers pointing forward. Practicing with blocks (on the lowest height) under your hands and the wall at your back can help make this pose more accessible. As you settle the weight of your torso onto your upper arms and squeeze your legs into your arms, lift the toes of one foot off the ground and then the other, any amount. As you practice over time, work toward straightening your legs as you balance. Return to a squat.

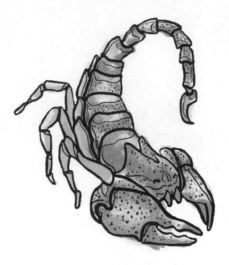

VRSCHIKASANA—SCORPION POSE

This pose also requires you to support the weight of your body on your arms. Kneeling on your hands and knees, drop your elbows down to where your palms were. You may also want to try facing a wall at first. Lift your hips up into what is often known as dolphin pose, a forearm variation of downward-facing dog. Begin to walk your toes toward your elbows, then raise one foot at a time into a forearm stand. Look forward at the ground between your hands. As you balance, arch your back and reach your feet toward the top of your head. To work up to this pose, practice dolphin at the wall and alternatively kick one foot at a time up and back to touch the wall. If you practice handstands already, you can try the variation of vrschikasana in which you support yourself on your palms instead of your forearms. Rest in child's pose when you come out of the balance.

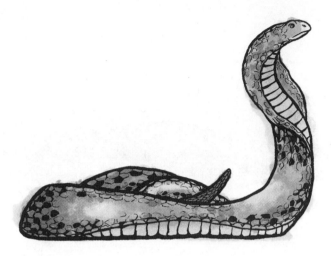

BHUJANGASANA—COBRA POSE

From downward-facing dog, scooch your toes back so you can drop your hips down and open your chest, looking slightly above eye level. Relax your hips, legs, and the tops of your feet to the ground. Let your elbows bend. Gently look to the left and the right, stretching your neck. Shed the support of your hands, hovering them above the ground, and maintain the backbend to any degree. Be armless and serpentine. Relax onto your belly on the floor with your right cheek down. Rise into cobra and then rest in between a few more times, remembering to breathe while bhujanga. From a chair, sit on the edge of the seat and arch your back, opening your chest. Reach your arms out from your shoulders and bend your elbows ninety degrees into "cactus arms."

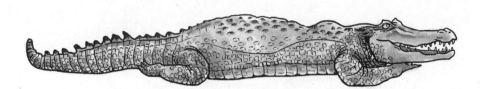

NAKRASANA—CROCODILE POSE

While on your belly on the ground, place your right hand on top of your left hand on the floor beneath your chin and relax your forehead on top of them. Space should remain underneath your shoulders while you relax them away from your ears and enjoy a stretch through the back of your neck. Home sweet home. Press up onto your hands and knees.

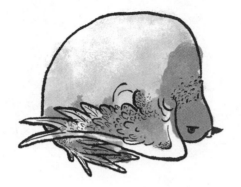

KAPOTASANA—PIGEON POSE

From kneeling in a table position, move your right knee behind your right wrist. Reach your left leg long behind you, placing a blanket underneath the knee and keeping the top of your foot flat on the floor. Then, carefully and gently move your right heel to underneath your left hip. With your palms open and down on the ground or on top of blocks, open up through your heart and floof your chest feathers. Gaze toward the sky. Relax your shoulders and keep your hips squarish. You can place another folded blanket under your right hip to keep from sinking on that side. To come out of the pose, slowly move your right knee back to meet the left and ease down onto your belly. For a softer pigeon experience, lay on your back, bend your left knee, and keep your left foot on the ground. Bend your right knee and place the outside of your right ankle above your left knee.

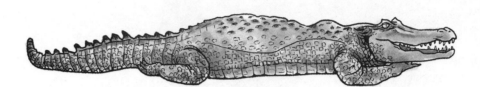

NAKRASANA—CROCODILE POSE

While on your belly on the ground, place your left hand on top of your right hand on the floor beneath your chin and relax your forehead on top of them. Check again that there is space underneath your shoulders. Breathe. You have always been home. Press up onto your hands and knees.

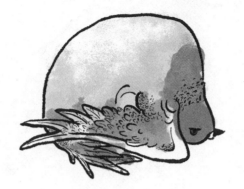

KAPOTASANA—PIGEON POSE

From kneeling in a table position, move your left knee behind your left wrist. Reach your right leg long behind you. Then, carefully and gently move your left heel underneath your right hip. Open your chest. Do the kapotasana shuffle. To come out of the pose, roll gently onto your left hip and come into a seated position.

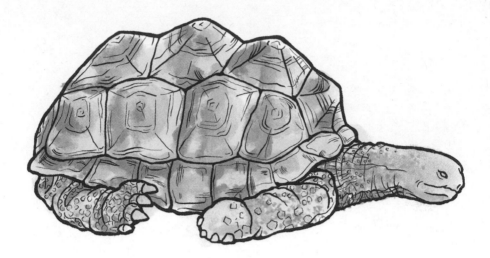

KURMASANA—TURTLE POSE

From a seated position, spread your legs as wide as is comfortable and bend your knees to create space under your legs. Hinge forward from your hips and inch your hands—any amount—underneath your legs. Relax your head and neck. Ponder a turtle story. For a more restorative experience, you can place rolled-up blankets underneath your knees and fold forward onto a tower of pillows or the soft seat of a chair. Relax your arms anywhere that is comfy. Coming close to the ground is not important. You simply want to feel the mental and emotional inward-turning that results from folding forward. Cover yourself with a blanket and brumate for a bit.

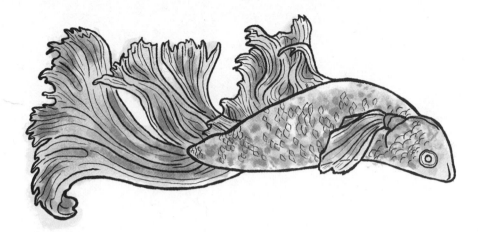

MATSYASANA—FISH POSE

Lie on your back. With straight arms, place your hands underneath your bottom, palms down, as you open your chest. Then, at the same time, lift your heart and shoulders, shift weight into your forearms, and let the crown of your head drop back to kiss the ground. You will likely feel stretching through the front of your body and in your throat. To experience a supported version of matsyasana, lie back on a couple of pillows or a bolster to support your torso and the back of your head. Let your shoulders "waterfall" off the sides of your props, opening your heart. Don't forget to breathe. You are a fish; you are the water itself.

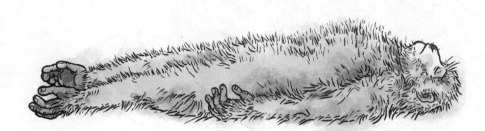

SAVASANA—CORPSE POSE

Dim the lights, put on your socks, and turn off any music. Sink into the support of the earth (or your mattress!) and rest there on your back, decomposing in unity with all the earth's beings. Use your props in any way you choose to ensure that you feel comfortable and supported. After twenty minutes or so, roll onto one side with your knees bent. Rest there for a minute or two more. Then, move slowly into any seated position. Bring your palms together in front of your heart. May you take your yoga from the mat into the wild world and treat all beings and yourself with compassion.

Acknowledgments

There are so many beings who made this book possible. Thank you to my writing group, the Wordy Birds: Cammie Fuller, Kris Jarvis, and Kirsten Dueck. To KT Hanson, saudaraku, the only gal I wanna sit on the beach and discuss multispecies entanglements with. To my editor, Shayna Keyles, and the rest of the wonderful folks at NAB—I couldn't imagine a more perfect fit for my first publishing experience.

I am e-turtle-y grateful to the following storytellers: Rachael Green, Jeffrey Popp, Danna Hinderle, and Jeannie Martin. To Luisa and Leandra, who got me through the worst of the eagle chapter and beyond—you give me hope whether I want it or not! Thanks to Dr. Sam Sheikali, Jen Cossette, Catie and Gerry Dutcher, Amy Moore, Eleanor Harris, Kristi Faull, my whole (P)EWCL fam, and all those who care for animals, captive and wild, and who inspire others to care for them too. Thank you tail-slaps to my beaver-believing dream team: Ross Fuller, Mo Cheikhali, Cathy Howard, and Aaron Hall. *Terima kasih* to Amir, Ical, and the Sulawesi farmers who shared stories and watermelon and laughter with me. Thank you to Libby Henrickson for teaching me cheetah pose, and to the other Open Book staff and customers who asked, "How's the writing going?"

Thank you to Annie Moyer for her feedback on the pose sequence, Pooja Virani for her review of select chapters, John Sherburne for help with Sanskrit terminology, and the entire Sun and Moon Yoga community who turned me into the yoga teacher and student that I am today. To my yoga students who endure animal noises and nature references with smiles and open hearts—I appreciate you (Ted Lasso style!). Additionally, I honor those who have taught all limbs of yoga throughout history, so these practices are available to us today. I acknowledge that most of this book was written on the ancestral lands of the Manahoac.

Deepest gratitude to the writers I admire so much, who offered endorsements and encouragement before I believed this book was worthy of it. And to all the nature writers who inspire me as they diversify and shape this genre for the better: Robin Wall Kimmerer, Joanna Macy, Aimee Nezhukumatathil, Temple Grandin, Richard Wagamese, Andrew Schelling, Sy Montgomery, J. Drew Lanham, and so many others. Thanks to Renee Askins who wrote the book, *Shadow Mountain*, that set me on this wild path.

Love to so many beyond-human beings: Meeko, Matsya, Monkey, Gus, Fiki, Denver, Taylor, Sprout, Eevee, Grover, Esssther, Danny, Siddhartha, Jim, Dwight, Bodhi, Shanti, Aladdin, Susu, the beavs, and countless, nameless others who made me who I am. Love to Hanuman, to the Goddess, and the mountains.

Finally, thank you is not nearly enough for Mom, Dad, Kev, Jordyn, and the rest of my amazing family from Florida to Hyderabad and places in between—your support makes the earth home. To Vishu—my most favorite animal of all—I love you.

Notes

INTRODUCTION

1 Darwin, C. *Origin of species variorum.* 1872, Darwin Online. 52.

2 De Waal, F. Are we in anthropodenial? *Discover,* 1997. **18**(7): 50–53.

3 Bennett, J. *Vibrant matter: A political ecology of things.* 2010, Durham, NC: Duke University Press.

4 Govindrajan, R. *Animal intimacies: Interspecies relatedness in India's Central Himalayas.* 2018, Chicago, IL: University of Chicago Press.

5 Cope, S. *Yoga and the quest for the true self.* 1999, New York, NY: Bantam Books. 77.

6 Cope, *Yoga and the quest for the true self.*

7 Satchidananda, S.S. *The yoga sutras of Patanjali.* 2012, Buckingham, VA: Integral Yoga Publications.

8 Barkataki, S. *Embrace yoga's roots: Courageous ways to deepen your yoga practice.* 2020, Orlando, FL: Ignite Yoga and Wellness Institute.

9 Tiwari, B.M. *The path of practice: A woman's book of Ayurvedic healing.* 2000, New York, NY: Ballantine Books. 71–72.

10 Mallinson, J. *The Gheranda Samhita: The original Sanskrit and an English translation.* 2004, Woodstock, NY: YogaVidya.com. 123.

11 Mallinson, *The Gheranda Samhita.* 16.

12 Mallinson, *The Gheranda Samhita.*

13 Barkataki, *Embrace yoga's roots.* 36.

14 Pattanaik, D. *Pashu: Animal tales from Hindu mythology.* 2014, London, UK: Penguin UK.

15 Pattanaik, D. *Pashu.*

16 Mitchell, S. *Bhagavad Gita: A new translation.* 2000, New York, NY: Three Rivers Press. 145.

17 Beasley, S.C. *Kindness for all creatures: Buddhist advice for compassionate animal care.* 2019, Boulder, CO: Shambhala Publications.

18 Schelling, A. *Wild form, savage grammar: Poetry, ecology, Asia.* 2003, Albuquerque, NM: La Alameda Press.

19 Hanh, T.N. *Zen and the art of saving the planet.* 2021, New York, NY: HarperCollins Publishers. 23–24.

20 Hanh, *Zen and the art of saving the planet.* 304.

21 Satchidananda, *The yoga sutras of Patanjali.*

22 Meloy, E. *Eating stone: Imagination and the loss of the wild.* 2005, New York, NY: Pantheon Books. 87.

23 Young, J., E. Haas, and E. McGown. *Coyote's guide to connecting with nature.* 2016, Shelton, WA: OWLLink Media.

24 Vitt, L.J., and J.P. Caldwell. *Herpetology: An introductory biology of amphibians and reptiles.* 2009, San Diego, CA: Elsevier Academic Press.

25 Ross, A., et al. National survey of yoga practitioners: Mental and physical health benefits. *Complementary Therapies in Medicine*, 2013. **21**(4): 313–323.

26 Cope, *Yoga and the quest for the true self.*

27 Cope, S. *The great work of your life: A guide for the journey to your true calling.* 2012, New York, NY: Random House USA Inc.

28 Barkataki, *Embrace yoga's roots.* 13.

29 De Waal, F. *Mama's last hug: Animal emotions and what they tell us about ourselves.* 2019, New York, NY: W.W. Norton & Company.

30 Mortali, M. *Rewilding: Meditations, practices, and skills for awakening in nature.* 2019, Boulder, CO: Sounds True. 106.

31 Kimmerer, R. *Braiding sweetgrass: Indigenous wisdom, scientific knowledge and the teachings of plants.* 2016, Minneapolis, MN: Milkweed Editions.

32 Bekoff, M. *Rewilding our hearts: Building pathways of compassion and coexistence.* 2014, Novato, CA: New World Library.

33 Johnson, M.C. *Skill in action: Radicalizing your yoga practice to create a just world.* 2017, Portland, OR: Radical Transformation Media.

CHAPTER 1: MATSYA—FISH

1 Gillespie, P.F. *Foxfire 7*. 1982, Garden City, NY: Anchor Books.

2 Hamidan, N. The freshwater fish fauna of Jordan. *Biologiezentrum Linz/Austria*, 2004. **2**: 385–394.

3 Loorz, V. *Church of the wild: How nature invites us into the sacred*. 2021, Minneapolis, MN: Augsburg Fortress Publishers. 59.

4 De Waal, F. *Mama's last hug: Animal emotions and what they tell us about ourselves*. 2019, New York, NY: W.W. Norton & Company.

5 Marris, E. *Wild souls: Freedom and flourishing in the non-human world*. 2021, New York, NY: Bloomsbury Publishing USA.

6 Balcombe, J. *What a fish knows: The inner lives of our underwater cousins*. 2016, New York, NY: Scientific American/Farrar, Straus and Giroux.

7 Balcombe, *What a fish knows*.

8 Balcombe, *What a fish knows*.

9 Balcombe, *What a fish knows*.

10 Aryasura. *Once the Buddha was a monkey: Arya Sura's Jatakamala*. 1989, Chicago, IL: University of Chicago Press. 103.

11 Hirschman, E.C. Consumers and their animal companions. *Journal of Consumer Research*, 1994. **20**(4): 616–632.

12 Bachman, N. *The language of yoga: Complete A-to-Y guide to asana names, Sanskrit terms, and chants*. 2004, Boulder, CO: Sounds True.

13 Safina, C. *Beyond words: What animals think and feel*. 2020, London, UK: Souvenir Press.

14 Safina, *Beyond words*; De Waal, F. *Are we smart enough to know how smart animals are?* 2016, New York, NY: W.W. Norton & Company.

15 Marris, *Wild souls*.

16 Balcombe, *What a fish knows*.

17 Balcombe, *What a fish knows*.

18 Marris, *Wild souls*.

19 Balcombe, *What a fish knows*.

20 Brammah, M. *The betta bible: The art and science of keeping bettas*. 2015, Martin Brammah.

21 Balcombe, *What a fish knows*.

22 Balcombe, *What a fish knows.*

23 Balcombe, *What a fish knows.* 208.

24 Stibbe, A. *Animals erased: Discourse, ecology, and reconnection with the natural world.* 2012, Middletown, CT: Wesleyan University Press.

25 Newkirk, I. Fish lessons, in *Kinship with the animals.* M. Tobias and K. Solisti-Mattelon, eds. 1998, Hillsboro, OR: Beyond Words Pub. 196.

26 Blau, T., and M. Blau. *Buddhist symbols.* 2004, New York, NY: Sterling.

27 Kaivalya, A., and A. Van der Kooij. *Myths of the asanas: The stories at the heart of the yoga tradition.* 2020, San Rafael, CA: Mandala Publishing.

28 Marris, *Wild souls.*

29 De Waal, *Mama's last hug;* Balcombe, *What a fish knows.*

30 De Waal, *Mama's last hug.*

31 De Waal, *Mama's last hug.*

32 De Waal, *Mama's last hug.*

33 De Waal, *Mama's last hug.*

34 Rosen, R. *The yoga of breath: A step-by-step guide to pranayama.* 2002, Boulder, CO: Shambhala Publications. 267.

35 Rosen, *The yoga of breath.*

CHAPTER 2: GARUDA—EAGLE

1 Carson, R. *Silent spring.* 1962, Boston, MA: Houghton Mifflin Company.

2 Chödrön, P. *When things fall apart: Heart advice for difficult times.* 1997, Boulder, CO: Shambhala Publications. 43.

3 Rosell, F., and R. Campbell-Palmer. *Beavers: Ecology, behaviour, conservation, and management.* 2022, Oxford, UK: Oxford University Press.

4 Starr, M. *Wild mercy: Living the fierce and tender wisdom of the women mystics.* 2019, Boulder, CO: Sounds True. 67.

5 Hellou, J., M. Lebeuf, and M. Rudi. Review on DDT and metabolites in birds and mammals of aquatic ecosystems. *Environmental Reviews,* 2013. **21**(1): 53–69.

6 King, B.J. *How animals grieve.* 2013, Chicago, IL: University of Chicago Press.

7 *Bald eagle life history.* All about Birds. 2019. www.allaboutbirds.org /guide/Bald_Eagle/lifehistory.

8 Pavlik, S., and W.B. Tsosie. *Navajo and the animal people: Native American traditional ecological knowledge and ethnozoology.* 2014, Golden, CO: Fulcrum Publishing.

9 NCTC Eagle Cam. U.S. Fish & Wildlife Service. Accessed July 7, 2022. www.fws.gov/office/national-conservation-training-center-facility /nctc-eagle-cam.

10 Mock, D.W., H. Drummond, and C.H. Stinson. Avian siblicide. *American Scientist*, 1990. **78**(5): 438–449.

11 Mortali, M. *Rewilding: Meditations, practices, and skills for awakening in nature.* 2019, Boulder, CO: Sounds True. 38.

12 Thompson, S. *Winterseer animal companion.* 2021, Woodbury, MN: Llewellyn Publications.

13 Pavlik and Tsosie, *Navajo and the animal people.*

14 Gahbler, N., and J. Macy. *Pass it on: Five stories that can change the world.* 2010, Berkeley, CA: Parallax Press.

15 Bachman, N. *The language of yoga: Complete A-to-Y guide to asana names, Sanskrit terms, and chants.* 2004, Boulder, CO: Sounds True.

16 Iyengar, B. *Light on yoga.* 1979, New York, NY: Schocken Books Inc.

17 Pattanaik, D. *Pashu: Animal tales from Hindu mythology.* 2014, London, UK: Penguin UK.

18 Pattanaik, *Pashu.* 246.

19 Davison, G.W.H., and H.Y. Fook. *A photographic guide to birds of Borneo.* 1996, Sanibel Island, FL: Ralph Curtis Books; Strange, M. *A photographic guide to the birds of Indonesia.* 2012, Tokyo, Japan: Tuttle Publishing.

20 Taylor, B. *Encyclopedia of religion and nature.* Vol. 1. 2008, New York, NY: Bloomsbury Publishing.

21 Solloway, K., and S. Stutzman. *The yoga anatomy coloring book: A visual guide to form, function, and movement.* 2018, New York, NY: Get Creative. 6.

22 Iyengar, *Light on yoga*; Brown, C. *Yoga bible: The definitive guide to yoga.* 2003, Cincinnati, OH: Walking Stick Press.

23 Kaivalya, A., and A. Van der Kooij. *Myths of the asanas: The stories at the heart of the yoga tradition.* 2020, San Rafael, CA: Mandala Publishing.

24 Schelling, A. *Wild form, savage grammar: Poetry, ecology, Asia.* 2003, Albuquerque, NM: La Alameda Press. 149.

25 Haupt, L.L. *Rooted: Life at the crossroads of science, nature, and spirit.* 2021, New York, NY: Little, Brown Spark. 36.

26 Haupt, *Rooted.* 36.

27 Kipfer, B.A. *Natural meditation: Refreshing your spirit through nature.* 2018, New York, NY: Skyhorse Publishing. 143.

28 NCTC Eagle Cam.

CHAPTER 3: KAPOTA—PIGEON

1 Stockton, S. *Meditations with cows: What I've learned from Daisy, the dairy cow who changed my life.* 2020, New York, NY: Penguin. 49.

2 Sibley, D. *The Sibley guide to birds.* 2000, New York, NY: Alfred A. Knopf.

3 Watanabe, S. Van Gogh, Chagall and pigeons: Picture discrimination in pigeons and humans. *Animal Cognition,* 2001. **4**(3): 147–151.

4 Sibley, *The Sibley guide to birds.*

5 Blanchan, N. *Bird neighbors: An introductory acquaintance with one hundred and fifty birds commonly found in the gardens, meadows, and woods about our homes.* 1904, New York, NY: Doubleday, Page & Co. 109.

6 Jerolmack, C. How pigeons became rats: The cultural-spatial logic of problem animals. *Social Problems,* 2008. **55**(1): 1.

7 Jerolmack, How pigeons became rats. 72.

8 Iyengar, B. *Light on yoga.* 1979, New York, NY: Schocken Books Inc. 367.

9 Brown, C. *Yoga bible: The definitive guide to yoga.* 2003, Cincinnati, OH: Walking Stick Press; Flynn, L. *Yoga for children: 200+ yoga poses, breathing exercises, and meditations for healthier, happier, more resilient children.* 2013, Avon, MA: Adams Media; Schiffmann, E. *Yoga: The spirit and practice of moving into stillness.* 1996, New York, NY: Pocket Books.

10 Leopold, A. On a monument to the pigeon in *A Sand County almanac.* 1966, New York, NY: Ballantine Books. 116.

11 Tolle, E. *The power of now: A guide to spiritual enlightenment.* 2004, Novato, CA: New World Library.

12 Mosco, R. *A pocket guide to pigeon watching: Getting to know the world's most misunderstood bird.* 2021, New York, NY: Workman Publishing. 7.

13 Le Page, J., and L. Le Page. *Mudras for healing and transformation.* 2nd ed. 2014, Sebastopol, CA: Integrative Yoga Therapy.

CHAPTER 4: BIDALA/GO—CAT/COW

1 Benanav, M. *Himalaya bound: One family's quest to save their animals—and an ancient way of life.* 2019, New York, NY: Simon and Schuster.

2 Govindrajan, R. *Animal intimacies: Interspecies relatedness in India's Central Himalayas.* 2018, Chicago, IL: University of Chicago Press. 50.

3 Stockton, S. *Meditations with cows: What I've learned from Daisy, the dairy cow who changed my life.* 2020, New York, NY: Penguin. 128.

4 Merriam, D. *The untold story of Sita: An empowering tale for our time.* 2020, New York, NY: SitaRam Press.

5 Dhanwatey, H.S., et al. Large carnivore attacks on humans in central India: A case study from the Tadoba-Andhari Tiger Reserve. *Oryx,* 2013. **47**(2): 221–227.

6 Roach, M. *Fuzz: When nature breaks the law.* 2021, New York, NY: W.W. Norton & Company.

7 Mishra, H., and J. Ottaway. *Bones of the tiger: Protecting the man-eaters of Nepal.* 2010, Guilford, CT: Lyons Press.

8 Acharya, K.P., et al. Human-wildlife conflicts in Nepal: Patterns of human fatalities and injuries caused by large mammals. *PLoS One,* 2016. **11**(9): e0161717; Lham, D., et al. Ecological determinants of livestock depredation by the snow leopard *Panthera uncia* in Bhutan. *Journal of Zoology,* 2021. **314**(4): 275–284; Wilkinson, C.E., et al. An ecological framework for contextualizing carnivore–livestock conflict. *Conservation Biology,* 2020. **34**(4): 854–867.

9 Jackson, R.M., and R. Wangchuk. A community-based approach to mitigating livestock depredation by snow leopards. *Human Dimensions of Wildlife,* 2004. **9**(4): 1–16.

10 Van Eeden, L., A. Treves, and E. Ritchie. Guardian dogs, fencing, and "fladry" protect livestock from carnivores. *The Conversation,* 2022. https://theconversation.com/guardian-dogs-fencing-and-fladry-protect-livestock-from-carnivores-103290.

11 Foltz, R. *Animals in Islamic tradition and Muslim cultures.* 2006, Oxford, UK: Oneworld. 94.

12 Schiffmann, E. *Yoga: The spirit and practice of moving into stillness.* 1996, New York, NY: Pocket Books.

13 Taylor, B. *Encyclopedia of religion and nature*. Vol. 1. 2008, New York, NY: Bloomsbury Publishing.

14 Serpell, J.A. Domestication and history of the cat. *The Domestic Cat: The Biology of Its Behaviour*, 2000. **2**: 180–192.

15 Young, R. *The secret life of cows*. 2017, London, UK: Penguin Books.

16 Fox, E. The Asian city obsessed with cats. *BBC Travel*, 2017. www.bbc .com/travel/article/20170531-the-asian-city-obsessed-with-cats.

17 Krishna, N. *Hinduism and nature*. 2017, Gurgaon, Haryana, India: Penguin Random House India Private Limited.

18 Pattanaik, D. *7 secrets of the goddess*. 2014, Chennai, India: Westland. 149.

19 Pattanaik, D. *Pashu: Animal tales from Hindu mythology*. 2014, London, UK: Penguin UK.

20 Pattanaik, *7 secrets of the goddess*. 115.

21 Singh, H., and L. Gibson. A conservation success story in the otherwise dire megafauna extinction crisis: The Asiatic lion (Panthera leo persica) of Gir forest. *Biological Conservation*, 2011. **144**(5): 1753–1757.

22 Walston, J., et al. Bringing the tiger back from the brink—the six percent solution. *PLoS Biology*, 2010. **8**(9): e1000485.

23 Jhala, Y., et al. Recovery of tigers in India: Critical introspection and potential lessons. *People and Nature*, 2021. **3**(2): 281–293.

24 Karanth, K.U. Saving the Indian tiger: Where do we go from here?, in *Voices in the wilderness: Contemporary wildlife writings*, P.S. Bindra, ed. 2010, New Delhi: Rupa & Co. 95–106.

25 Pattanaik, *Pashu*.

26 Reinhardt, V., and A. Reinhardt. Cohesive relationships in a cattle herd (Bos indicus). *Behaviour*, 1981. **77**(3): 121–151.

27 Stranger than fiction—A leopard and motherly cow. *On Forest*. 2014. www.onforest.com/forest/stranger-than-fiction-a-leopard-and -motherly-cow.

28 Giggs, R. Cows need friends to be happy. *The Atlantic*, November 2019.

29 Pitt, D., et al. Domestication of cattle: Two or three events? *Evolutionary Applications*, 2019. **12**(1): 123–136.

30 Kluever, B.M., et al. Vigilance in cattle: The influence of predation, social interactions, and environmental factors. *Rangeland Ecology and Management*, 2008. **61**(3): 321–328.

31 Pattanaik, *Pashu*.

32 Rabinowitz, A. *Chasing the dragon's tail: The struggle to save Thailand's wild cats*. 2002, Washington, DC: Island Press.

33 Mortali, M. *Rewilding: Meditations, practices, and skills for awakening in nature*. 2019, Boulder, CO: Sounds True. 70.

34 Haupt, L.L. *Rooted: Life at the crossroads of science, nature, and spirit*. 2021, New York, NY: Little, Brown Spark. 192.

CHAPTER 5: TITTIBHA—FIREFLY

1 Nezhukumatathil, A. *World of wonders: In praise of fireflies, whale sharks, and other astonishments*. 2020, Minneapolis, MN: Milkweed Editions.

2 Constantz, G. *Hollows, peepers, and highlanders: An Appalachian mountain ecology*. 2nd ed. 2004, Morgantown, WV: West Virginia University Press.

3 Constantz, *Hollows, peepers, and highlanders*.

4 Nezhukumatathil, *World of wonders*.

5 Constantz, *Hollows, peepers, and highlanders*.

6 Constantz, *Hollows, peepers, and highlanders*.

7 Constantz, *Hollows, peepers, and highlanders*.

8 Constantz, *Hollows, peepers, and highlanders*.

9 Brown, C. *Yoga bible: The definitive guide to yoga*. 2003, Cincinnati, OH: Walking Stick Press.

10 Constantz, *Hollows, peepers, and highlanders*. 77.

CHAPTER 6: BHUJANGA—SERPENT

1 Covington, D. *Salvation on Sand Mountain: Snake handling and redemption in southern Appalachia*. 1995, New York, NY: Penguin. 177.

2 Burnett, J. Snake-handling preachers open up about "takin' up serpents." National Public Radio online, October 4, 2013; accessed

October 19, 2022. http://archive.kuow.org/post/snake-handling -preachers-open-about-takin-serpents.

3 Burnett, J. Serpent experts try to demystify Pentecostal snake handling. National Public Radio online, October 18, 2013; accessed October 19, 2022. www.npr.org/2013/10/18/236997513/serpent-experts-try -to-demystify-pentecostal-snake-handling.

4 Wilcox, C. *Venomous: How Earth's deadliest creatures mastered biochemistry*. 2016, New York, NY: Scientific American/Farrar, Straus and Giroux.

5 Pattanaik, D. *Pashu: Animal tales from Hindu mythology*. 2014, London, UK: Penguin UK.

6 Lasater, J.H. *30 essential yoga poses: For beginning students and their teachers*. 2003, Berkeley, CA: Rodmell Press. 97.

7 Lasater, *30 essential yoga poses*.

8 Kaivalya, A., and A. Van der Kooij. *Myths of the asanas: The stories at the heart of the yoga tradition*. 2020, San Rafael, CA: Mandala Publishing.

9 Iyengar, B. *Light on yoga*. 1979, New York, NY: Schocken Books Inc. 107.

10 Solloway, K., and S. Stutzman. *The yoga anatomy coloring book: A visual guide to form, function, and movement*. 2018, New York, NY: Get Creative. 6.

11 Lasater, *30 essential yoga poses*.

12 Moore, Amy. Introducing Esther: PVAS's Snake Ambassador. Potomac Valley Audubon Society Valley Views newsletter, 2021. **40**(2): 6–7.

13 Red Cornsnake. Virginia Herpetological Society, 2022. www.virginia herpetologicalsociety.com/reptiles/snakes/corn-snake/corn_snake.php.

14 Steen, D.A. *Secrets of snakes: The science beyond the myths*. 2019, College Station, TX: Texas A&M University Press. 81.

15 McAdory, P. How my pet snake taught me to really see. *New York Times* online, December 28, 2020; accessed October 19, 2022. www.nytimes .com/2020/12/28/magazine/pet-snakes.html.

16 Bachman, N. *The language of yoga: Complete A-to-Y guide to asana names, Sanskrit terms, and chants*. 2004, Boulder, CO: Sounds True.

17 Pattanaik, D., and Tulsidasa. *Wisdom of the gods for you and me: My Gita and my Hanuman Chalisa*. 2019, New Delhi: Rupa. 320.

18 Khalsa, S.K. *Kundalini yoga as taught by Yogi Bhajan: Unlock your inner potential through life-changing exercise.* 2000, London, UK: DK Books.

19 Khalsa, G.K., and C. Michon. *The eight human talents: Restore the balance and serenity within you with Kundalini yoga.* 2000, New York, NY: Harper.

20 Satchidananda, S.S *The yoga sutras of Patanjali.* 2012, Buckingham, VA: Integral Yoga Publications. 77.

CHAPTER 7: HANUMAN—MONKEY

1 Seyfarth, R.M., D.L. Cheney, and P. Marler. Vervet monkey alarm calls: Semantic communication in a free-ranging primate. *Animal Behaviour,* 1980. **28**(4): 1070–1094.

2 Safina, C. *Beyond words: What animals think and feel.* 2020, London, UK: Souvenir Press.

3 Safina, *Beyond words.*

4 Smuts, B. Encounters with animal minds. *Journal of Consciousness Studies,* 2001. **8**(5–7): 293–309.

5 Recio, B. *Inside animal hearts and minds: Bears that count, goats that surf, and other true stories of animal intelligence and emotion.* 2017, New York, NY: Skyhorse Publishing.

6 Vanamali. *Hanuman: The devotion and power of the monkey god.* 2010, Rochester, VT and Toronto, CAN: Inner Traditions; Bedi, A. *Gods and goddesses of India.* 1998: Eshwar.

7 Pattanaik, D., and Tulsidasa. *Wisdom of the gods for you and me: My Gita and my Hanuman Chalisa.* 2019, New Delhi: Rupa. 320.

8 Pattanaik and Tulsidasa, *Wisdom of the gods for you and me.*

9 Wolfe, L.D. Rhesus macaques: A comparative study of two sites, Jaipur, India, and Silver Springs, Florida, in *Primates face to face: The conservation implications of human-nonhuman primate interconnections,* A. Fuentes and L. Wolfe, eds. 2002, Cambridge, UK: Cambridge University Press.

10 Wolfe, *Rhesus macaques.*

11 Vanamali, *Hanuman.*

12 Pattanaik and Tulsidasa, *Wisdom of the gods for you and me.*

13 Vanamali, *Hanuman.*

14 Vanamali, *Hanuman.*

15 Iyengar, B. *Light on yoga.* 1979, New York, NY: Schocken Books Inc.

16 Pattanaik and Tulsidasa, *Wisdom of the gods for you and me.*

17 Schiffmann, E. *Yoga: The spirit and practice of moving into stillness.* 1996, New York, NY: Pocket Books.

18 Kaivalya, A., and A. Van der Kooij. *Myths of the asanas: The stories at the heart of the yoga tradition.* 2020, San Rafael, CA: Mandala Publishing.

19 Kaivalya and Van der Kooij, *Myths of the asanas.*

CHAPTER 8: VRSCHIKA—SCORPION

1 Daley, J. Slo-Mo footage shows how scorpions strike. *Smithsonian.* April 6, 2017.

2 Wilcox, C. *Venomous: How Earth's deadliest creatures mastered biochemistry.* 2016, New York, NY: Scientific American/Farrar, Straus and Giroux.

3 Wilcox, *Venomous.* 23.

4 Wilcox, *Venomous.*

5 Wilcox, *Venomous.*

6 Wilcox, *Venomous.*

7 Wilcox, *Venomous.*

8 Wilcox, *Venomous.*

9 Benton, T. Reproduction and parental care in the scorpion, *Euscorpius flavicaudis. Behaviour,* 1993. **117**(1–2): 20–28.

10 Courtship. *Micro monsters with David Attenborough.* 2013. Season 1, Episode 3.

11 Brown, C.A., and D.R. Formanowicz. Reproductive investment in two species of scorpion, *Vaejovis waueri (Vaejovidae)* and *Diplocentrus linda (Diplocentridae),* from west Texas. *Annals of the Entomological Society of America,* 1996. **89**(1): 41–46.

12 Ugolini, A., and M. Vannini. Parental care and larval survival in *Euscorpius carpathicus. Italian Journal of Zoology,* 1992. **59**(4): 443–446.

13 Gaffin, D.D., et al. Scorpion fluorescence and reaction to light. *Animal Behaviour,* 2012. **83**(2): 429–436.

14 Wilcox, *Venomous.*

15 Wolf, H. Scorpions' pectines—idiosyncratic chemo- and mechano-sensory organs. *Arthropod Structure & Development,* 2017. **46**(6): 753–764.

16 Iyengar, B. *Light on yoga.* 1979, New York, NY: Schocken Books Inc.

17 Iyengar, *Light on yoga.* 388.

18 Loorz, V. *Church of the wild: How nature invites us into the sacred.* 2021, Minneapolis, MN: Augsburg Fortress Publishers.

19 Hanh, T.N. Thich Nhat Hanh on walking meditation. *Lion's Roar.* February 18, 2022. www.lionsroar.com/how-to-meditate-thich-nhat-hanh-on-walking-meditation.

CHAPTER 9: NAKRA—CROCODILE

1 Webb, G.J., S.C. Manolis, and M.L. Brien. Saltwater crocodile *Crocodylus porosus,* in *Crocodiles. Status survey and conservation action plan.* S.C. Manolis and C. Stevenson, eds. 3rd ed. 2010, Darwin, NT, Australia: Crocodile Specialist Group. 99–113.

2 Platt, S., et al. Frugivory and seed dispersal by crocodilians: An overlooked form of saurochory? *Journal of Zoology,* 2013. **291**(2): 87–99.

3 Fitzner, Z. *Tears for crocodilia: Evolution, ecology, and the disappearance of one of the world's most ancient animals.* 2022, Yardley, PA: Westholme Publishing LLC.

4 Garrick, L.D., J.W. Lang, and H.A. Herzog. Social signals of adult American alligators. *Bulletin of the AMNH,* 1978. **160**(3): 153–192.

5 Ouchley, K. *American alligator: Ancient predator in the modern world.* 2013, Gainesville, FL: University Press of Florida; Swiman, E., et al. *Living with alligators: A Florida reality.* 2005, Gainesville, FL: University of Florida/IFAS.

6 Swiman, et al., *Living with alligators.*

7 Fitzner, *Tears for crocodilia.* 131.

8 Fitzner, *Tears for crocodilia.* 180.

9 Ouchley, *American alligator.*

10 Elder, E. Menacing alligator, almost 12 feet long, killed in Silver River by state-licensed trapper. *Ocala Star Banner,* March 10, 2022.

11 Ouchley, *American alligator.*

12 Swiman, et al., *Living with alligators.*

13 Ouchley, *American alligator.*

14 Fitzner, *Tears for crocodilia.*

15 Swiman, et al., *Living with alligators.*

16 Fitzner, *Tears for crocodilia.*

17 Fitzner, *Tears for crocodilia.* 51.

18 Behler, J., and D. Behler. *Alligators and crocodiles.* 1998, Stillwater, MN: Voyageur Press.

19 Fitzner, *Tears for crocodilia.*

20 Behler and Behler, *Alligators and crocodiles.*

21 Behler and Behler, *Alligators and crocodiles.*

22 Brown, C. *Yoga bible: The definitive guide to yoga.* 2003, Cincinnati, OH: Walking Stick Press.

23 Fitzner, *Tears for crocodilia.*

24 Fitzner, *Tears for crocodilia.*

25 Fitzner, *Tears for crocodilia.*

26 Ogden, L.A. *Swamplife: People, gators, and mangroves entangled in the Everglades.* 2011, Minneapolis, MN: University of Minnesota Press.

27 Burton, R. *The Marjorie.* 2022. https://themarjorie.org.

28 Carrico, E.K. *The other side of the river: Stories of women, water, and the world.* 2015, Shanagarry, Cork, Ireland: Womancraft Publishing. 74.

CHAPTER 10: USTRA—CAMEL

1 Adams, C. *Camel crazy: A quest for miracles in the mysterious world of camels.* 2019, Novato, CA: New World Library.

2 Schiffmann, E. *Yoga: The spirit and practice of moving into stillness.* 1996, New York, NY: Pocket Books.

3 Iqbal, A., and B.B. Khan. Feeding behaviour of camel. Review. *Pakistan Journal of Agricultural Sciences,* 2001. **38**: 58–63.

4 Kingsolver, B. *How to fly (in ten thousand easy lessons).* 2020, New York, NY: Harper.

5 Adams, *Camel crazy.*

6 Reading, R.P., et al. Wild Bactrian camel conservation. *Exploration into the Biological Resources of Mongolia,* 2005. **9:** 91–100.

7 Myers, L.R. *The joy of knitting: Texture, color, design, and the global knitting circle.* 2001, Philadelphia, PA: Running Press.

8 Loorz, V. *Church of the wild: How nature invites us into the sacred.* 2021, Minneapolis, MN: Augsburg Fortress Publishers.

9 Adams, *Camel crazy.*

10 Parkes, Clara. *The knitter's book of yarn: The ultimate guide to choosing, using, and enjoying yarn.* 2007, New York: NY: Potter Craft.

11 Kingsolver, *How to fly.*

12 Adams, *Camel crazy.*

13 De Waal, F. *Mama's last hug: Animal emotions and what they tell us about ourselves.* 2019, New York, NY: W.W. Norton & Company.

14 al-Tirmidhi, J. Tie it and rely (upon Allah). July 10, 2022. https://sunnah.com/tirmidhi:2517.

15 Adams, *Camel crazy.*

16 Alhadrami, G., and B. Faye. Camel. *Encyclopedia of Dairy Sciences,* 2022. **1:** 48–64.

17 Faye, B. The camel, new challenges for a sustainable development. *Tropical Animal Health and Production,* 2016. **48**(4): 689.

18 Lokhit Pashu-Palak Sansthan. *Saving the camel and peoples' livelihoods: Building a multi-stakeholder platform for the conservation of the camel in Rajasthan.* 2005, Proceedings of an International Conference held on 23–25 November 2004 in Sadri, Rajasthan, India; Foltz, R. *Animals in Islamic tradition and Muslim cultures.* 2006, Oxford, UK: Oneworld.

19 Adams, *Camel crazy.*

20 Ruurs, M. *My librarian is a camel: How books are brought to children around the world.* 2005, Honesdale, PA: Astra Publishing House.

21 Kipling, R., and L. Zwerger. *How the camel got his hump.* 2001, New York, NY: North-South Books.

22 Adams, *Camel crazy.*

23 Lokhit Pashu-Palak Sansthan, *Saving the camel and peoples' livelihoods.*

24 Iqbal and Khan, Feeding behaviour of camel.

25 Faye, The camel, new challenges for a sustainable development.

26 Faye, The camel, new challenges for a sustainable development; Ahmad, S., et al. Economic importance of camel: Unique alternative under crisis. *Pakistan Veterinary Journal,* 2010. **30**(4): 191–197.

27 Sansthan, *Saving the camel and peoples' livelihoods.*

28 Whitley, H.L. Forget the reindeer, holidays at Mount Vernon feature a different kind of furry friend. *Southern Living* online, December 21, 2020.

29 Douglas-Klotz, N. *The Sufi book of life: 99 pathways of the heart for the modern dervish.* 2005, New York, NY: Penguin. 257–258.

30 Laws, J.M., and E. Lygren. *The Laws guide to nature drawing and journaling.* 2016, Berkeley, CA: Heyday. 3.

CHAPTER 11: ŚVANA—DOG

1 Schleidt, W.M., and M.D. Shalter. Co-evolution of humans and canids: An alternative view of dog domestication. *Evolution and Cognition,* 2003. **9**: 57–72.

2 Yong, E. A new origin story for dogs. *The Atlantic,* June 2016. 2.

3 Tsing, A. Unruly edges: Mushrooms as companion species. *Environmental Humanities,* 2012. **1**: 141.

4 Starr, M. *Saint Francis of Assisi: Brother of creation.* 2013, Boulder, CO: Sounds True.

5 Kotler, S. *A small furry prayer: Dog rescue and the meaning of life.* 2010, New York, NY: Bloomsbury Publishing USA.

6 De Waal, F. *Mama's last hug: Animal emotions and what they tell us about ourselves.* 2019, New York, NY: W.W. Norton & Company.

7 Kotler, *A small furry prayer.* 251.

8 Paquet, P.C., and L.N. Carbyn. Gray wolf: *Canis lupus* and allies, in *Wild mammals of North America: Biology, management, and conservation,* G.A. Feldhamer, B.C. Thompson, and J.A. Chapman, eds. 2003, Baltimore, MD: Johns Hopkins University Press. 482–510.

9 Flores, D. *Coyote America: A natural and supernatural history.* 2016, New York, NY: Basic Books. 16.

10 Senani, K. Wild dogs, in *Nature chronicles of India*, A. Banerjee, ed. 2014, New Delhi: Rupa. 16.

11 Pavlik, S., and W.B. Tsosie. *Navajo and the animal people: Native American traditional ecological knowledge and ethnozoology.* 2014, Golden, CO: Fulcrum Publishing.

12 Louv, R. *Our wild calling: How connecting with animals can transform our lives—and save theirs.* 2019, Chapel Hill, NC: Algonquin Books.

13 Mitchell, B.R., M.M. Jaeger, and R.H. Barrett. Coyote depredation management: Current methods and research needs. *Wildlife Society Bulletin,* 2004. **32**(4): 1209–1218.

14 Timm, R.M., et al. Coyote attacks: An increasing suburban problem. University of California, Davis: Hopland Research and Extension Center, 2004.

15 Flores, *Coyote America.*

16 Alexander, S.M., and D.L. Draper. Worldviews and coexistence with coyotes, in *Human-wildlife interactions.* B. Frank, J.A. Glikman, and S. Marchini, eds. 2019, Cambridge, UK: Cambridge Univesity Press. 311–334.

17 Flores, *Coyote America,* 148.

18 Flores, *Coyote America.*

19 Nilep, C. "Code switching" in sociocultural linguistics. *Colorado Research in Linguistics,* 2006. **19**: 1–21.

20 Harmon-Jones, E., and J. Mills. An introduction to cognitive dissonance theory and an overview of current perspectives on the theory. *Cognitive Dissonance: Progress on a Pivotal Theory in Social Psychology,* 2019. 3–24. https://doi.org/10.1037/0000135-001.

21 Lasater, J.H. *30 essential yoga poses: For beginning students and their teachers.* 2003, Berkeley, CA: Rodmell Press. 67.

22 Schiffmann, E. *Yoga: The spirit and practice of moving into stillness.* 1996, New York, NY: Pocket Books. 118.

23 Brown, C. *Yoga bible: The definitive guide to yoga.* 2003, Cincinnati, OH: Walking Stick Press.

24 Bekoff, M. Social play in coyotes, wolves, and dogs. *Bioscience,* 1974. **24**(4): 225–230.

25 *Coyote and badger: More friendship (and waddles) in extended video—California Wildlife Camera.* 2020. https://youtu.be/mGyHlYPupHg.

26 Dell'Amore, C. Why this coyote and badger "friendship" has excited scientists. *National Geographic* online. February 5, 2020. www.nationalgeographic.com/animals/article/coyote-badger-video-behavior-friends#:~:text=Research%20has%20backed%20up%20the,and%20stalk%20Uinta%20ground%20squirrels.

27 Satchidananda, S.S. *The yoga sutras of Patanjali.* 2012, Buckingham, VA: Integral Yoga Publications. 8.

28 Louv, *Our wild calling.* 109.

29 Kotler, *A small furry prayer.* 258.

30 Estes, C.P. *Women who run with the wolves: Myths and stories of the wild woman archetype.* 1995, New York, NY: Ballantine Books. 20.

CHAPTER 12: KURMA—TORTOISE/TURTLE

1 Tobias, M., and K. Solisti-Mattelon. *Kinship with the animals.* 1998, Hillsboro, OR: Beyond Words. 126.

2 Frazer, S.J.G. *The golden bough.* 1966, London, UK: Macmillan.

3 Kimmerer, R. *Braiding sweetgrass: Indigenous wisdom, scientific knowledge and the teachings of plants.* 2016, Minneapolis, MN: Milkweed Editions.

4 Laufer, P. *Dreaming in turtle: A journey through the passion, profit, and peril of our most coveted prehistoric creatures.* 2018, New York, NY: St. Martin's Press. 9.

5 Roach, M. *Fuzz: When nature breaks the law.* 2021, New York, NY: W.W. Norton & Company. 149.

6 Tobias and Solisti-Mattelon, *Kinship with the animals.* 21.

7 Laufer, *Dreaming in turtle.* 20.

8 Laufer, *Dreaming in turtle.* 51.

9 Carr, A. *Handbook of turtles: The turtles of the United States, Canada, and Baja California.* 1952, Ithaca, NY: Cornell University Press. 143.

10 Iyengar, B. *Light on yoga.* 1979, New York, NY: Schocken Books Inc. 292.

11 Iyengar, *Light on yoga.*

12 Tobias and Solisti-Mattelon, *Kinship with the animals.* 22.

13 Mitchell, S. *Bhagavad Gita: A new translation*. 2000, New York, NY: Three Rivers Press. 57.

14 Mattison, C. *Firefly encyclopedia of reptiles and amphibians*. 2015, Buffalo, NY: Firefly Books.

15 Tobias and Solisti-Mattelon, *Kinship with the animals*. 127.

16 DiNardo, K., and A.P. Hayden. *Living the sutras: A guide to yoga wisdom beyond the mat*. 2018, Boulder, CO: Shambhala.

17 Iyengar, B. *Light on life: The yoga journey to wholeness, inner peace, and ultimate freedom*. 2005: Rodale. 12–13.

18 Mattison, *Firefly encyclopedia of reptiles and amphibians*.

19 King, B.J. *How animals grieve*. 2013, Chicago, IL: University of Chicago Press.

20 Tobias and Solisti-Mattelon, *Kinship with the animals*. 22.

CHAPTER 13: SAVA—CORPSE

1 Li, T., et al. Maternal responses to dead infants in Yunnan snub-nosed monkey *(Rhinopithecus bieti)* in the Baimaxueshan Nature Reserve, Yunnan, China. *Primates,* 2012. **53**(2): 127–132.

2 Huang, Z.-P., et al. The use of camera traps to identify the set of scavengers preying on the carcass of a golden snub-nosed monkey *(Rhinopithecus roxellana)*. *PLoS One,* 2014. **9**(2): e87318.

3 Holzmann, I., et al. Impact of yellow fever outbreaks on two howler monkey species *(Alouatta guariba clamitans* and *A. caraya)* in Misiones, Argentina. *American Journal of Primatology,* 2010. **72**(6): 475–480.

4 Appiah-Opoku, S. Indigenous beliefs and environmental stewardship: A rural Ghana experience. *Journal of Cultural Geography,* 2007. **24**(2): 79–98.

5 Haupt, L.L. *Rooted: Life at the crossroads of science, nature, and spirit*. 2021, New York, NY: Little, Brown Spark. 74.

6 Lasater, J.H. *Yoga myths: What you need to learn and unlearn for a safe and healthy yoga practice*. 2020, Boulder, CO: Shambhala.

7 Pattanaik, D. *Sita: An illustrated retelling of the Ramayana*. 2013, London, UK: Penguin UK.

8 Goswami, T. *Ramacaritamanasa/The Hindu Bible*. 2017, Middletown, DE: Only RAMA Only.

9 Goswami, *Ramacaritamanasa/The Hindu Bible*.

10 Ogada, D.L., F. Keesing, and M.Z. Virani. Dropping dead: Causes and consequences of vulture population declines worldwide. *Annals of the New York Academy of Sciences*, 2012. **1249**(1): 57–71.

11 Ogada, Keesing, and Virani, Dropping dead.

12 Bhusal, K.P., I.P. Chaudhary, and D.B. Rana. Vultures and people: Some insights into an ancient relationship and practice of sky burial persisting in trans-Himalayan region of Nepal. *Vulture Bulletin*, 2020. **9**: 43–45.

13 Barkataki, S. *Embrace yoga's roots: Courageous ways to deepen your yoga practice*. 2020, Orlando, FL: Ignite Yoga and Wellness Institute. 174.

14 Elbroch, M., and C. McFarland. *Mammal tracks & sign: A guide to North American species*. 2019, Guilford, CT: Stackpole Books.

15 Govindrajan, R. *Animal intimacies: Interspecies relatedness in India's Central Himalayas*. 2018, Chicago, IL: University of Chicago Press. 22.

16 Roach, M. *Fuzz: When nature breaks the law*. 2021, New York, NY: W.W. Norton & Company. 139.

17 Haraway, D.J. *Staying with the trouble: Making kin in the Chthulucene*. 2016, Durham, NC: Duke University Press.

CONCLUSION: TADASANA—MOUNTAIN POSE

1 Leopold, A. *A Sand County almanac*. 1966, New York, NY: Ballantine Books. 137.

2 Thoreau, H.D. Walking. *The Atlantic* online archives. June 1862; accessed October 19, 2022. www.theatlantic.com/magazine/archive/1862/06/walking/304674.

3 Askins, R. *Shadow mountain: A memoir of wolves, a woman, and the wild*. 2002, New York, NY: Anchor.

Index

D

E

About the Author

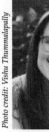

ALISON ZAK is a writer, yoga teacher, wildlife conservationist, and founder and director of the Human–Beaver Coexistence Fund. She lives in Virginia with her husband and a few more beloved furry, feathery, and finny beings. This is her first book. Learn more at www.alisonzak.com and follow her on Instagram and Twitter @animal_asana.

About North Atlantic Books

North Atlantic Books (NAB) is an independent, nonprofit publisher committed to a bold exploration of the relationships between mind, body, spirit, and nature. Founded in 1974, NAB aims to nurture a holistic view of the arts, sciences, humanities, and healing. To make a donation or to learn more about our books, authors, events, and newsletter, please visit www.northatlanticbooks.com.